HOW WE AGE

HOW WE AGE

A DOCTOR'S JOURNEY
INTO THE HEART
OF GROWING OLD

Marc E. Agronin, M.D.

Da Capo Press
A Member of the Perseus Books Group

Designed by Pauline Brown
Set in 11.75 point AGaramond by the Perseus Books Group

Library of Congress Cataloging-in-Publication Data

Agronin, Marc E.
    How we age : a doctor's journey into the heart of growing old / Marc E.
Agronin.—1st Da Capo Press ed.
       p.   cm.
    Includes bibliographical references.
    ISBN 978-0-306-81853-0 (hardcover : alk. paper)
    ISBN 978-0-7382-1415-3 (e-book)
    1. Older people. 2. Nursing home patients—Florida—Miami. 3. Geriatric
psychiatry. 4. Aging. I. Title.
HQ1061.A485   2011
305.26—dc22
                                                            2010044261

Published by Da Capo Press
A Member of the Perseus Books Group
www.dacapopress.com

Da Capo Press books are available at special discounts for bulk purchases in the
U.S. by corporations, institutions, and other organizations. For more information,
please contact the Special Markets Department at the Perseus Books Group, 2300
Chestnut Street, Suite 200, Philadelphia, PA 19103, or call (800) 810-4145, ext.
5000, or e-mail special.markets@perseusbooks.com.

10 9 8 7 6 5 4 3 2 1

*To my beloved grandparents—the elders who
came before me and gave me a true appreciation
for growing old—Eva, Simon, Etta, and Tany*

CONTENTS

❊❊❊

Part IV
Wisdom

Part V
A Million Sparks

A Note to the Reader

It is with some trepidation that I have chosen to write about the lives of several individuals in this book. There is the risk that the retelling of a life, especially from the vantage point of a doctor, will not only fall short but will also end up trivializing certain aspects. There is the greater risk that stories of medical or psychiatric ailments end up dehumanizing the patient, portraying him or her as a disease and not as a human being.

My purpose in this book is to talk about aging by describing the lives of several individuals in a manner as humane and respectful as possible. To this end, I have retained the actual names of certain individuals with their permission only and have changed both the names and certain identifying biographical details of others so as to render them wholly anonymous. In several instances I created a composite of two similar individuals in order to retain the basic condition without allowing identification even by those who as clinicians or caregivers knew these individuals personally. Finally, there are several individuals portrayed in this book whose deaths have made it impossible to obtain permission. In those instances I have again changed names and other details to preserve anonymity. My sincere hope is that these efforts have yielded a work that respects and even extols its subjects.

Introduction

For nearly every doctor, the very first encounter in medical school with an old person is with a corpse. I discovered this fact on the first day of gross anatomy class when our instructors led us up to the dissection lab and introduced us to the rows of human cadavers that would serve as our teachers and companions for the next six months. Everyone was a little uneasy that morning, and I welcomed the nervous glances and smiles of classmates as we filtered through the room searching for what we hoped would be the perfect body. "Look for a thin woman," my labmates Steve and Jimmy each whispered to me, recalling the sage advice of an older classmate trying to steer us toward an easier dissection experience. "Who can tell?" I shot back, staring out at the dozen black slate tables in the room, topped off with human forms wrapped in heavy white gauze and covered with translucent plastic sheets. I reasoned to my labmates that it was like trying to find King Tut among a room full of mummies, and so we quickly abandoned our original plan and went for a table near the window. Even in the few short minutes we had spent in the room, the fumes of the formalin solution used to preserve the bodies were overpowering, and so I hoped that at least an open window would provide some respite from the smell.

"Please help your labmates remove the plastic coverings on your cadaver," the professor called out, "and then strip off all of the gauze to expose the entire body." A shudder went through my own body, and I cringed. The entire body? "Yes, the entire body," the instructor continued, as if she were reading my mind, "and then pick it up and flip it over—get a good look." This was surely a technique not meant to teach as much as to flood our psyches with the glory of gross anatomy, dispensing all mystery and anxiety in one fell baptism of formalin. Entering the room had been unsettling enough, but at least then the cadavers had been covered. I had honestly never seen a dead body before and was hoping to put off the experience as long as possible. But within minutes I was surrounded by teams of sweating medical students piling up strips of smelly, greasy gauze and struggling to pick up rigid and very heavy formalin-logged bodies. I remember one particularly surreal moment as I watched four classmates bearing the strangest of grins as they hoisted the cadaver off the table, grunting at its weight and struggling to grip the slippery, leathery skin.

The unmasking of the face of our cadaver unnerved me the most. I had hoped in vain to skip that altogether and heed the words of the second anatomy instructor, who was strutting through the room and cautioning against removing too much gauze so as not to dry out the body. He argued gruffly with the first instructor that her shock treatment was unnecessary, finally shouting, "If they can't stand looking at the body, they shouldn't be in medicine!" My labmates were more obedient to the initial instructions and summarily removed the plastic bag from the head and began to unravel the gauze. I stood back and envisioned seeing what archaeologists had discovered in the mummified faces of pharaohs—coal-black visages with bony physiognomy and time-scorched skin that resembled cracked china. Those ancient, royal faces looked more skeletal than human and lacked all of the machinery of expression that might have betrayed a final emotion.

When the last strip of gauze was peeled away, I looked down on the face of our cadaver, mesmerized by her silent, still expression, her upper cheek muscles and eyelids slightly scrunched as if a puff of air had been blown into her face at the moment of death. The face appeared inert, like a totem permanently carved into clay or stone and so different from the blushing, breathing face of a living person. And yet this had been a person, I realized, who once had walked the earth and lived a life like everyone else in the room—working, loving, running, eating, perhaps bearing and raising children. Although the identities of and any biographical information about the cadavers used in medical school anatomy courses are never revealed to the students, the unmasking of our cadaver revealed numerous deep facial wrinkles and a few thin strands of silver hair matted on her head that betrayed one critical fact: She had been quite *old* when she died. We later learned that she had been ninety-eight at the time of her death from a heart attack.

After we rewrapped the head and limbs of the cadaver, the dissection of the torso began in earnest, initiated by a brief instructional paragraph in the course manual: "Palpate bony landmarks on cadaver: clavicle, jugular notch, sternal angle, sternum. . . . Incise skin from jugular notch to 3 cm above the pubic symphysis in mid-line cutting around the umbilicus. . . . Then incise superficial fascia." These instructions sounded straightforward, but they underestimated the magnitude of the task. We did not merely "incise" superficial fascia (the elastic connective tissue that covers and supports the muscles), but we cut, slit, ripped, pulled, melted, and gushed it all over instruments, hands, table, and cadaver, all while we were constricted by two to three layers of gloves and heavy blue smocks.

If we were exceedingly careful and dexterous, the dissection proceeded smoothly over the ensuing months and actually taught us, as budding doctors, some human anatomy—even though a living patient is wholly unlike a cadaver in color, form, and feel. But for the average student, the time spent with the chopped and tattered remains of the cadaver cast a certain spell of nonchalance and banality over behaviors that would otherwise have been deemed inappropriate and even atrocious. One cadaver in our lab, for example, wore a pair of plastic Groucho Marx glasses throughout the course. Another cadaver in the room was decked out one morning with a party hat, balloons, and a sign that read, "Happy Birthday" for the celebrating student. And there were worse examples.

But what struck me most from the very beginning of gross anatomy was how the ninety-eight-year-old "she" lying before me was repeatedly designated an "it," a mere object to be manipulated, incised, cracked open, and explored throughout the dissection process. And this is where gross anatomy began to change from a respectful and educational part of the medical school curriculum into a dehumanizing rite of passage, what eminent cardiologist and Nobel Prize winner Dr. Bernard Lown calls a "grievous error" as a way to start off medical training. He goes on to deride the "denaturing of human values" that follows when students come to view the "repulsive formaldehyded body being dissected as an inanimate object, forgetting that it was once a fellow human being."

Lown's perspective hit me acutely one evening when I had been assigned to bring home the "bone box," a small hinged maple coffin that carried the ossified and disassembled remains of some poor soul. The bone box was meant to afford the student a more intimate educational communion with a human skeleton: a time to study the intricacies of each bone, to search for the hidden grooves where ligaments and tendons anchor themselves, and to palpate the angles and contours of the shafts and joints. Of course, the bearer of the bone box was also the subject of much, well, ribbing from other students, who warned of the midnight knocking and clacking that might emanate from the box. By that point in the course I thought I was inured to any such jibing and imaginings, but the box sat uneasily beneath my bed. I contemplated the bones and wondered whose form they had once supported. "Alas, poor Yorick!" I imagined a ghostly Hamlet cry as he cradled his jester's skull, "I knew him. . . . / Here hung those lips that I have kiss'd I know not how oft." William Shakespeare understood well the transformation from being to bone:

Imperious Caesar, dead and turn'd to clay,
Might stop a hole to keep the wind away:
O, that that earth, which kept the world in awe,
Should patch a wall to expel the winter flaw!

So too, these dry bones resting beneath the springs of my cot would remain the permanent dry relics of an unknown soul. There would be no prophetic cry from Ezekiel to God to bind them back together, to layer on muscle, sinew, and flesh and have them walk the earth again, resuming whatever holy or unholy tasks this person had once engaged in.

Over the months of gross anatomy the old woman who lay on our slate table slowly disintegrated, torn apart bit by bit until the final coup de grâce at course end: "Make a midsagittal cut completely through the entire head and neck. Leave the nasal septum attached intact to one side of the split head by cutting the septum free from the palate and skull."

From the very first day of gross anatomy, I had dreaded this lab, having already read the last page of the course manual, just as many people do with a good mystery. I was horrified then by the instructions, and yet when the time came, I found myself fearlessly and robotically sawing through the skull and neck and splitting the two halves of the head from each other. With the brain and skullcap already removed and most of the face and neck cut away, what remained looked only remotely human. This final lesson ended the course unceremoniously, and we all fled the lab, relieved to finally be free from the stink of the formalin. But a lesson on the meaning and end result of aging had been imprinted indelibly on our delicate doctor psyches.

That lesson learned in the first few months of medical training and reinforced in nearly every other experience was unmistakable: *Aging equals death*. Every course throughout the next few years, from pathology to physiology, and then to clinical work on the wards, focused on how the workings of the body could go awry. From a young doctor's vantage point, the aging process brought only decay, decline, and disease until the inevitable demise of the body. This depressing view of aging, reinforced during my years of internship and residency in medicine, neurology, and psychiatry, was then coupled with a new equation: *Aging equals dementia* (the brain disease that robs people of memory and other parts of their intelligence).

This second aging equation was represented by a common derogatory term I heard used to describe older demented patients: "gomer." I am not certain of the etymology of this word, but it was popularized by Samuel Shem's famous novel *The House of God*, a book about medical internship that has been read often by every frustrated, overworked, and cynical doctor-in-training since the book's publication in 1978. Shem's character the "Fat Man" serves as a wise but crass senior resident and mentor for neophyte hospital interns, and he introduces them to the world of gomers on day one: "'Gomer is an acronym: Get Out of My Emergency Room—it's what you want to say when one's sent in from the nursing home at 3 A.M. . . . But gomers are not just dear old people,' said Fats. 'Gomers are human beings who have lost what goes into being human beings. They want to die, and we will not let them. We're cruel to the gomers, by saving them, and they're cruel to us, by fighting tooth and nail against our trying to save them. They hurt us, we hurt them.'"

During training I discovered that these so-called gomers (or "gomes," for short) were ubiquitous figures in every medical setting. They were individuals with Alzheimer's disease or other forms of dementia who were permanently disoriented and unable to effectively communicate, care for themselves, and control their behaviors. On psychiatric wards my compatriots further nicknamed a subset of the gomes the "shriekers and smearers," inspired by episodes of blood-curdling screams or the throwing or smearing of feces that were viewed as repulsive and completely off the rails of rational human behavior. The primary care doctors and geriatricians who attended to them in nursing homes were typically referred to as "gome-docs" and dismissed as either incompetent or overly sentimental individuals who couldn't hack more illustrious or challenging medical specialties.

This perceived equating of aging with death and aging with dementia represents a pervasive societal view that stigmatizes the elderly and denigrates the individuals who tend to them. These equations are the core premises of what noted gerontologist Robert Butler first called "ageism." And they have a basis in what we all see as the undeniable truths—indeed, the defining aspects—of aging. Our bodies change irrevocably and not, it seems, for the better. We see our most beloved ones suffer from illness, frailty, and loss. Skin pales and droops. Hair becomes brittle and colorless. Voices quiver and fade. Muscles wither. And personalities who once worked a trade, soldiered in battle, or mothered a beloved child falter and fade with time. *Parents age and die.*

In response to these "grim years of debilitation and disease with which most people's lives currently end," biogerontologist

Aubrey de Grey and a small wave of researchers contend that science should be able to find a cure for aging. In this model, age is a disease that warrants treatment. And for some entrepreneurial individuals who lack both the patience and the scientific acumen of de Grey and simply want some part of the fountain of youth, aging is also an economic opportunity. Witness the rise of the multi-billion-dollar industry of antiaging products and clinics. Whether it is a costly wrinkle cream, a deluxe series of hormone shots, or a facelift, a growing number of people are willing to pay top dollar for such treatments. Many of my colleagues are less sanguine about reversing the effects of aging and focus instead on promoting a triad of physical exercise, healthy diet, and mentally stimulating activities to preserve both intellect and physical strength as long as possible.

To the extent that we think about the inevitability of aging and death, we usually have great trepidation—a sentiment captured well by Psalm 71:9: "Do not cast me off in old age; when my strength fails, do not forsake me." Face-to-face encounters with older individuals force us to look momentarily into an eternal abyss and trigger unanswerable questions about life and death that can bring wonder as easily as fear and despair. For the young doctor, the antidotes to these fears are corpse and gome—dehumanized bodies that the doctor can easily poke, cut, and crack open without a lot of emotion. When reduced to objects, the aged don't seem so bad, we reason, because *they* are not *us*. For the rest of society, there are many other ways to dehumanize the elderly and hide from what gerontologist Lars Tornstam aptly labels age-centric perceptions of the "nuisances and miseries" of old age.

✠✠✠

For many months after completing the gross anatomy course, I continued to wrestle with my experiences of working with a dead person. I would hearken back to a particularly vivid memory from class when the dissection required the corpses to be sitting upright on the slate table. Despite a somewhat human pose, everything sacred about both the body and its persona seemed stripped off the cadaver. Any small fantasies or fears of rejuvenation or zombification of the body that I still harbored by that point in the class faded away completely, and I said to myself, "There's no coming back." I now understood what the words "from dust to dust" meant. But this understanding did not bring satisfaction. I was particularly worried about how my growing lack of sensitivity toward the corpse could easily creep one step back to the extremely debilitated, aged patient. The two seemed, at times, to merge into one. I asked myself, "How does a doctor—how does anyone, for that matter—maintain a positive regard toward aging while simultaneously having to witness the loss, suffering, and utter degradation that it brings?"

I have learned since then that these dismal equations of aging with decrepitude along with the rigid and defensive attitudes that they inspire are only one side of the story. The other side is too often overlooked in our dread of aging. This realization first came to me several months after completing gross anatomy when I began volunteering at a nursing home down the street from the medical school. I was assigned to visit Esther, a one-hundred-year-old woman who, I must admit, looked uncannily like the cadaver I had just spent the previous six months with! Surprisingly, this realization was not eerie but comforting. And Esther could not have been more of a delight to be with. Her mind and wit were sharp, she smiled constantly, and she reveled in our time together. One day she described to me in detail the births of her three children, then extended their life stories over decades to the present. One moment I was hearing about her beloved young children, and the next moment I was meeting them in person—then in their seventies! There were many moments when I closed my eyes and simply listened to Esther, losing track of the nearly eighty years between us. And I began to see age in a different context: Someone living with the daily infirmities of aging and approaching death could still enjoy most of the same human experiences we find so precious in younger years. Unfortunately, we often fail to see these positive elements in the lives of our elders because we are so focused on the physical or mental decline of aging. The body will certainly reach its limits, with death beyond our ability to predict or control. But the true failure here is not old age; rather, it is the failure of our own creativity and willingness to conceive that life up until its last moments has its own ways and meanings.

In the spring of my second year in medical school, Esther died several weeks after suffering a stroke. During our last visit she struggled to talk and reach out to me despite the loss of speech wrought by a small clot in her brain. As with so many of the older patients with whom I had grown close over the years, I had put the possibility of her death out of my mind, imagining that she was actually my own age but just looked a little different. In fact, I have often employed such mental gymnastics to deal with aging and death in my own family. Shortly after my grand-parents passed away, I compressed much of my grief into an odd fantasy that in the afterlife they had moved down to Miami Beach and were experiencing eternal bliss together, with endless sunny beaches and Early Bird Specials. Florida, I imagined, was actually some form of Shangri-La where all of our deceased eld-erly could be found happily wandering around if we just looked hard enough.

As fate would have it, I currently live and work in Miami as a doctor for old people—the very profession so derided in my early years of training. In this location, I frequently encounter several unique groups of elders, including aged Holocaust sur-vivors and Cuban exiles, who have exerted a disproportionate influence on my clinical work and have inspired so much of my writing. To be more specific, I am the psychiatrist at the Miami Jewish Health Systems, the site of one of the largest nursing homes in the United States. Although people sometimes call my place of work "God's waiting room," they miss a much big-ger picture. True, the average age of my patients is about ninety years old, meaning that I see a lot of people close to one hundred. The eighty-year-olds who come to see me are like teenagers on my scale of things and the seventy-year-olds—babies! And true, my job is to tend to all of the maladies and infirmities of aging. But as I first learned from Esther and then from countless others, the true scales of aging are not one-sided; the problems of aging must be weighed against the promises. In my work as a geriatric psychiatrist I have learned that *aging equals vitality, wisdom, cre-ativity, spirit,* and, ultimately, *hope.* And for an increasing number of aged individuals, these vital forces are growing by the day.

❈❈❈

My mission in this book is to offer a more balanced perspective on aging. My intention is not to promise any cures for aging, as some books do. I am not interested in pushing certain nutritional supplements, diets, or lifestyles as fountains of youth, as other books try. I am interested solely in honestly exploring the experience of old age through the lives of my patients. I begin in Part I by defining the aging process as it is currently understood scientifically and as it is imagined and experienced psychologically. Part II is a medical rounds of sorts in which I describe the aging process of several of my most memorable patients. These cases, though quite variable in their life stories, illustrate clearly the inevitable physical, psychological, and social changes that make aging such a challenge and bring us ever closer to the end of living. Each story, in its own way, also shows the many promises of aging that transform both the ways in which our bodies and brain age and the experience of aging itself.

Part III discusses the changing role of memory in old age, telling some surprising stories of how life persists and even thrives in the face of memory loss. Part IV looks at the meaning and development of wisdom and how it is practiced by our elders— as well as by the caregivers for these elders. In both parts I highlight several sages who exemplify all that is right about aging. In Part V, I extend the discussion of aging to the very frontiers of life, exploring how certain lessons learned from the aged can serve as beacons for all of us as we head into those very same waters. These lessons promise not the end of aging, but a new beginning even as we continue to age.

Part I
What Is Old?

Age I must, but die I would rather not.

—JOHN UPDIKE, "ENDPOINT"

Heaven
Can't Wait

The old woman had drawn down the shade in her room, trying, I imagined, to stop the midday Miami sun from penetrating her grief. But the sun still hit the window full force and illuminated the shade like a Chinese lantern. She sat silently in a wheelchair, her ninety-three-year-old silhouette appearing sad and stooped in the bathing light. I entered, held her hand for a moment, and introduced myself. "Sit down, Doctor," she said politely. I asked her why she had come to the nursing home, and she described the recent passing of her husband after seventy-three years of marriage. I was overwhelmed by the thought of her loss and wanted to offer some words of comfort. I leaned in close and spoke, "I'm so sorry. What has it been like for you losing your husband after so many years of marriage?" She paused for a moment and then replied, "Heaven."

I flinched at her answer, hoping that I had misheard her. Seeing my bewilderment and understanding immediately the irony of her response, she smiled at me and proceeded to describe how she had endured decades in an unhappy marriage with a gruff, verbally abusive man. As she spoke, I realized how my instincts were so completely off. In my misguided empathy, I had committed what William James describes as the psychologist's fallacy—assuming incorrectly to know what someone else is experiencing.

With this newly widowed patient, I imagined that only a life of sadness and decrepitude remained, and I felt badly about it. But I was wrong. She had not fallen into the abyss. Rather, she was glad to have finally won a measure of freedom and was determined to make the best of it. As her life unfolded at the nursing home over the next year, she threw herself into new activities and relationships in a way that was quite unexpected to me.

All of us lapse into such mistaken impressions of old age from time to time. Our mistake stems in part from an age-centric perspective in which we view our own age as the most normal of times, regarding it as representative of how all life should be. At eighteen the fifty-year-olds may seem ancient, but at fifty we are apt to say the same about the eighty-year-olds. So what's it really like to be old? I often query my patients, who are mostly in their late eighties and nineties, and the responses are surprising. "I forgot I was so old," a one-hundred-year-old patient recently told me and then excused herself to make it to bingo on time.

This age-centrism is particularly pervasive when we gauge attitudes toward nursing homes. All too often we imagine that life stops at the doors of a facility, that the life within, if we can call it that, is loveless and lonely, with death hovering close by. We make this mistake when we refuse to see needs for intimacy even in the most debilitated elderly. Our youth-centered culture equates love with sex, but I have seen with my older patients that love can be an endlessly blossoming flower, felt and expressed in hundreds of ways. A friend's mother who suffers from Alzheimer's disease has fallen in love with another resident on her floor, and they walk around holding hands and snuggling with a newfound innocence that perhaps only their memory loss restored.

We also project our terror of death onto the aged, assuming that fear and depression must stalk the final years of life. And yet in my fifteen years of working in nursing homes, I have never heard a patient tell me that he or she was afraid of death. Sometimes there is acceptance, other times anticipation, but most often there is no great concern. Life goes on in death's shadows.

In the end there is a cost to our myopic views of aging in which only the negative images appear. We imagine the pains of late-life ailments but not the joys of new pursuits; we recoil at the losses and loneliness and fail to embrace the wisdom and meaning that only age can bring. Henry Wadsworth Longfellow captured the sentiment well:

> For age is opportunity no less,
> Than youth itself, though in another dress,
> And as the evening twilight fades away,
> The sky is filled with stars, invisible by day.

This perspective on age, filled with both curiosity and optimism, is unfortunately not the norm. In general, we understand little about aging, and what we perceive is too often a
projection of our own fears. I am certain this is why I am often
challenged with two specific questions when I reveal that I am
a doctor for the elderly. The first question is, "What does it
mean to be old?" The second question flows from the first: "Is
it depressing to work with old people?" I could make it easy on
myself and simply answer, "It depends," and "No," but in reality
each question has a thousand different answers. "It's a gift," I
might answer to the first question on some days or "a tragedy"
on others. To the second question, I could confess to occasionally
feeling depressed, but in truth with each patient I have a different
state of mind—delight, disappointment, curiosity, consternation,
wonder. And with both questions, I always remind myself and
my questioners that I am merely an observer of age and not a
member of the aged—at least not yet. Nevertheless, these questions are profound, and my answers demand some deeper ex-
planations. Let me begin with an ending.

※※※

In the spring of 1997 my beloved grandfather passed away. A
week before his death, I stood vigil at his bedside while he flick-
ered between confusion and insensibility. The once-brilliant
mind of this retired doctor was soaked in a pool of morphine,
and most rational thinking had already drowned. He insisted
on wearing a large pair of sunglasses in the darkened room. He
cursed and growled when I held his arms as he staggered into

the bathroom. I am not certain that he even recognized me on that final visit, as by then his lifelong persona had largely separated from the person. Nevertheless, his voice came to me as I watched him lying in bed, breathing slowly: "Notice the abnormal rate and pitch of the breath sounds," I imagined him saying; "they are quiet at first but become increasingly labored until they stop for a moment—called *apnea*—and then the pattern repeats. This is known as Cheyne-Stokes respiration, and it is often seen just prior to death." I pictured the seriousness of my grandfather's face as he taught me to observe the ebb and flow of the respirations and then quizzed me to make certain that I had absorbed the lesson. The distinctive cadence of his voice alternated between curt instructions and impatient pauses, waiting for my answer. He had a way of repetitively flipping his outstretched hand at the wrist as he spoke, one finger extending out like Michelangelo's God, as if to say, "It can be this way, or that, but you must choose one!"

The practice of medicine was his life, and he had taught me with both an earnestness and a severity about caring for patients. My grandfather had experienced the urgency of his work while serving as a field surgeon in the U.S. Army Air Corps stationed on Okinawa during World War II. This sensibility was reinforced after the war in his fifty years as a general practitioner in the small industrial town of Kaukauna, Wisconsin. In both circumstances the survival of a patient depended on his own wit and hands; there were few colleagues or other resources to help out.

My grandfather had an instinctive sense of independence, no doubt fashioned in his childhood. He was born in 1914 and grew up in a small town in Ukraine near Kiev, alone with his mother and grandmother after his father left for America. He survived the poverty and deprivation of rural Russia during World War I and recalled hiding in haystacks or in the forest to escape from the murderous pogroms of the Cossacks. At the age of twelve he came to America in the steerage of a transatlantic steamer, landing at Ellis Island with other similarly huddled masses. My grandfather remembered seeing the gleaming torch of the Statue of Liberty as the ship glided into New York harbor. He remembered the sweet, precious taste of an orange that he ate, for the first time, while on board. His subsequent journey in America slowly took him west along the rail-lines; he lived with relatives in New York, Chicago, Madison, and, finally, Appleton, Wisconsin.

If you picture Wisconsin like the shape of a hand, Appleton is a small city located in the fleshy crook just below the thumb. It is the largest of a group of smaller towns and villages—including Kaukauna—that sit astride a shallow valley that hugs the bends and locks of the Fox River as it meanders from Lake Winnebago to Green Bay. The area is both picturesque and pastoral, surrounded by farms and woods, but with belching, steaming stacks of paper mills lying at its center. It was settled throughout the 1800s mainly by Dutch and German immigrants—farmers, dairymen, craftsmen, and small businessmen—but was no stranger to the small groups of itinerant German, Polish, and Russian Jews who found their way into its folds, including both sets of my great-grandparents.

My grandfather's father was a garrulous, backslapping businessman who ran a successful dairy and in the process befriended most of the city officials in Appleton, including a then-obscure judge named Joseph McCarthy. To his three sons, however, my great-grandfather was a firm and exacting father who fostered a competition among them better suited to the survival-of-the-fittest mentality of czarist Russia than to the open spirit of small-town America. My great-grandmother, in contrast, was a very bright and beloved woman with a good sense of humor, but she carried with her a sadness that she hadn't been able to leave behind in Russia. She was actually the first old person in my life, and I remember her as an exotic and perfumed lady with long painted fingernails, a mysterious accent, and a thick purple coat and scarf surrounding her wrinkled and wizened face. She was a babushka in purple.

Before becoming a doctor, my grandfather was, in succession, a milkman, a boxer, and a scientist. His appearance lent itself to each job, as he had the quick, thin legs of a deliveryman; the box-shaped, muscular trunk of a pugilist; and the round, balding, and bespectacled face of an intellectual. Photographs of him from youth to old age always show a dapper man, whether dressed in uniform, scrubs, or coat and tie. In 1938 he married my grandmother, and they stayed together for life. She was the consummate doctor's wife, who raised their three children, managed the books, and kept the home quiet, kosher, and revolving smoothly around his frenetic schedule.

As a doctor my grandfather worried incessantly about his patients, but he hid it behind his obsessive work habits and sometimes-gruff demeanor. He had a bad habit of throwing instruments during surgery when the wrong one was handed to him. He demanded perfection in himself, and he was relentless with his staff. By the early 1970s probably half of Kaukauna's residents were either current or former patients, a good many of them having been birthed into his hands. Neighbors, strangers, and family alike all made visits to his modest-sized, spartan clinic, where he was renowned as a diagnostician. There weren't many secrets in our large extended family living throughout Wisconsin, but whatever they were, he knew and kept them hidden as a good doctor should.

His perseverance and dedication were legendary. For example, several weeks after my grandfather's death, a former patient wrote a letter to the editor of the local newspaper to relate this story. One night during a fierce Wisconsin blizzard, the man's young daughter woke up with a high fever. He called my grandfather, who initially advised him to bundle her up and meet him at his office. Several minutes later the man's phone rang: "Stay home," my grandfather advised; "I will come to you." And as the man described, "In a time that only a man with purpose could make, there was a knock on the door and there stood a snowman." My grandfather entered, shook off the snow, and remained with the family throughout the night, tending to the man's beloved firstborn daughter. Many years later the man stood with that same daughter to watch her husband graduate from medical school. After the ceremony he pulled the new doctor aside and challenged him to repay the family's debt to my grandfather by embodying the same dedication to his craft.

Until the year before his death, aging had been a relatively benign process for my grandfather. He practiced medicine and surgery until the age of eighty and then retired not because he felt any desire to but because it just seemed logical. He played tennis, traveled, and even made a pilgrimage back to Ellis Island to see the same great hall in which he had been processed some sixty-eight years earlier. A perpetual student, he audited courses in neuroscience and German at nearby Lawrence University. I was in medical school at the time, and he would sometimes call me to discuss the role of a certain neurotransmitter or region of the brain that he was studying. He also spent his retirement tending to and doctoring my grandmother, saving her life on one occasion when her heart rate slowed precipitously.

When he became ill, however, aging caught up to him quite quickly. In the summer of 1996 he was diagnosed with an aggressive form of prostate cancer. I was called to Kaukauna immediately to offer him moral support—at a time when I was treating similarly aged and ill war veterans during my geriatric psychiatry training at the Minneapolis VA hospital. I had hoped that he would brush off the cancer like he had done with a small stroke a few years back, but within months it was clear that this would not be the case. Suddenly, he needed me for support and advice, and we spoke nearly every day about how to manage some of his physical discomfort. Of course, as a newly minted psychiatrist I was of little value to his medical management, and I left that up to my uncle, who had taken over his practice. But our conversations were not really about my grandfather's pain; they were, it seemed to me, cover for dealing with aging and death.

As the de facto family historian I also knew that I had to record his life stories, and so at Thanksgiving we sat down on the porch of my grandparents' house for a taped interview. The life review was almost too painful for him, however, and he broke down crying at several points. I had never seen him cry before, let alone show sadness, but I persisted with the camera, knowing that time was short. In my work with older individuals it is always painful to witness the crumbling of their composure in the face of loss and grief, but I can steel my own emotions because I rarely know what the person was once like. But such was not the case with my grandfather, and I vacillated between denial and despair. As I was saying my good-byes and leaving my grandparents' home at the end of the weekend, he pulled me aside and stated rather perfunctorily that this was probably the last time I would see him. His words were sterile and clinical—a doctor's way of parting with a patient. But I knew that this was his best effort at saying good-bye. A doctor myself, I brushed off his words in the same manner I might use leaving the clinic at day's end —"No, Grandpa; I'll see you soon. Call me tomorrow."

I reflected on these moments as I sat at his bedside that spring and tried to contain my emotions. He was not only my grandfather, but also my mentor, my inspiration, and, from my earliest childhood days, my own doctor. But now his life of eighty-three years was drawing to a close, and I was standing witness at the point where aging meets death. No other period of life has such a feared and mysterious ending. Childhood ends with the budding of puberty and the new challenges of adolescence. Adolescence passes away in the excitement of pulsating hormones, shedding its awkward, uncertain skin in the journey into young adulthood. The subsequent stages of adulthood bring undiscovered treasures of love, children, work, and spirit. Even in the face of failure or lost opportunities, there is always hope for something new. But aging seems to bring this process to a halt. The horizon is unknown except for the single fact that a true ending will come.

Even as my grandfather was slipping away, for me he was already changing from a presence to a memory and from a companion to a silent guide. But what I risked missing at the time was the same lesson I had learned several years earlier from my one-hundred-year-old friend, Esther—that aging is not synonymous with death. As I now contemplate the immensity of his influence on my own life, I realize that it wasn't his death but his old age that left such an imprint on me. Aging bequeathed him virtues of experience, vitality, and wisdom, but it was, in the end, simply his presence that made all the difference for me. In our last few months together I discovered what most of us instinctively know: that the primal answer to the question "What does it mean to be old?" is a beloved parent, grandparent, or other older figure.

The experiences and images of "oldness" that we absorb from aged people are immediately biased by the particulars of those people in our lives. The elders who populated my own childhood were all active, colorful, and beloved figures who conferred a delightful mystique on aging. This is why I have always felt comfortable working with the elderly. But not everyone has such vital figures in her or his life, and oldness may instead be a decrepit and mute grandfather in a wheelchair or an agitated aunt with dementia. The resultant vision of aging may be full of dread and even disgust. As I begin to answer the questions of age and refract the answers through the eyes of my many patients, I recognize that the stories capture only a piece of aging—not its entirety. But they're at least a good beginning.

Age I Must

Awareness of the difference in age between ourselves and our older caretakers is perhaps the first lesson of aging that we absorb. I am here in time and they are *there*, with there being some amorphous point farther along the timeline. At the age of four my youngest son, Sam, first made this connection, which led inevitably to some rather profound questions about age. At the time he was just beginning to count things in earnest, and what had started a year before as a show of fingers now began to flow onto objects in the environment. With each birthday came the announcement of a new age, and before long both time and space were taking on meaning as measurable dimensions. I wasn't prepared, though, for his youthful interrogation one morning.

Sam's questions began before I was fully awake and thus sufficiently attentive to his pressing curiosity. "Dad . . . do you work with old people?" he asked me. "Yes," I murmured from beneath the pillow. "Dad . . . do you *like* working with old people?" "Yes," I murmured again, still half-asleep. "Every day?" "Of course, Sam." "Even Tuesday?" "Yes, even Tuesday," I answered, again in a somnolent monotone. He paused for a minute, and I began to drift off. "Dad . . . are they just waiting to die?" This question landed like a shattered glass, and my eyes opened wide. I sat up. "Sam, why do you ask?" Even at four years old, it seemed, he had already absorbed this notion that aging somehow equaled death. He stared at me with a serene curiosity, smiling, but intent on an answer. Fortunately, his questions were coming faster than the answers I was searching for. "What is old?" he started in again, "and in how many days will I be old?"

This was a counting that I could not do for him, but the question fired my own curiosity about what being old is all about. As a doctor I measure it by years: Seventy years old has different expectations than ninety, and once you get beyond one hundred, it appears to be a whole new realm. But these distinctions, I realize, can be misleading. And they are changing by the day. At some point we see and feel changes in our minds and bodies that begin to define being old, and we ask the same questions posed by my son: What does it mean to grow old? When does old begin? And what does it entail?

For more complete answers than I could give my son, I must turn to scientists who have devoted their lives to the study of aging. One of these experts was preeminent geriatric psychiatrist Dr. Gene Cohen, who served as the head of the Center for Aging and Humanities at George Washington University. In 2009 I

spent an idyllic summer morning talking to him on the large
porch of his home in a quiet, wooded suburb of Washington,
DC. I questioned him about aging as my own son had questioned me. In response, he began with a story from his adolescence about a fish called the longhorn sculpin.

The longhorn sculpin is not a fish you'll ever find on a plate.
It's a rather ugly fish with a bulbous head, large protruding eyes,
and a thin brown and olive green body that tapers to a tailfin
under a phalanx of spines. For the fishermen who work the
shallow coastal waters of New England, the sculpin is a nuisance
because it eats up the bait intended for other fish and makes
a growling noise when handled. But for Cohen, the longhorn
sculpin was his entry into the study of aging. As a sixteen-
year-old high school student in 1960, he developed a new technique to determine the fish's age by using a small bone in its
inner ear called the otolith. When the otolith is snapped perfectly
in half, its inner accretions of calcium can be read like the rings
of a tree. Growing up in a small town south of Boston, Cohen
was able to use a newly invented minisaw at the nearby Woods
Hole Oceanographic Institute to accomplish this task for the
first time ever. He used these measurements to create a database
of growth norms for the sculpin and won first prize in a prestigious science fair for his project.

But it wasn't the award that inspired him so much as the
way in which he imagined aging to address larger issues. Knowing the age of the fish became a way of assessing the health of
the fish's habitat, which in turn allowed an exploration of even
wider issues—fish stocks, overfishing, ocean currents, and pol-
lution. For many years, however, the study of aging was like the

longhorn sculpin of scientific research, both neglected and more of a nuisance compared to other, more glamorous areas of research. And yet Cohen saw how the accumulating knowledge about aging applied to many other areas. For example, discoveries about how normal cells age and die have provided a doorway into understanding why cancerous cells don't.

Over the four decades of his career, the study of aging took Cohen in many different directions. But in response to my central question, he was clear: "Aging, of course, has two paths," he told me; "there's the process and there's the people." The process tells us how and why we age and is limited by laws of physics and biology. The people, however, show us how to age, and the limits are more variable. On the one hand, the experience of aging is circumscribed by physical health, personal resources, cultural norms, and historical events that are often out of our control. On the other hand, our own efforts can bring change and meaning to the aging process that can transcend these forces in ways that biology can't.

※※※

Several months after my conversation with Gene, I traveled from Miami to a large psychiatric conference in Las Vegas to deliver a talk on psychotherapy with elderly patients. As the plane crossed over the southwestern United States, I was lost in thought, pondering not the meaning of old but the breadth and beauty of the landscape below as the Grand Canyon came into view. I have discovered that it is impossible to capture the immensity of the Grand Canyon through the window of an airplane. On more than one occasion I have tried, from the confines of my seat, to snap a meaningful photograph of those sinuous cracks as they emerge and deepen in the flat desert earth below. The result is always disappointing, as the aerial vista of the canyon is just too vast and hazy amid the clouds at 37,000 feet. To really apprehend the Grand Canyon means standing right on it and then wandering down the serpentine trails carved beneath its rim. From that vantage point the profound depths of the canyon and its dazzling multilayered earthen colors emerge.

The Grand Canyon is a perfect illustration of how aging is a process of perpetual change. For the geologist, the passage of time can be seen in its ancient walls, with each epoch containing its own strata of rich colors and collections of fossils and other debris. Over millions of years the Colorado River carved away the earth and stone while the tectonic plate below lifted up an entire plateau and tilted it toward the southern rim, eventually yielding a stunning edifice. Like an old man or woman, the parched and stone-wrinkled body of the canyon stretches across the plateau, twisting and turning in the bedrock of schist and granite like an arthritic skeleton and sloughing off fossilized mollusks and corals from its sand-and-mudstone skin. The canyon was already an ancient being when the aboriginal Pueblo people first crept along its limestone spine and ribs and descended into its petrified innards. Its walls are sturdy in some places, crumbling in others, and wear an impressive timeworn face that easily distracts from the teeming wildlife on its ledges or within the impenetrable bowers of willow and brush that hug the edges of the river and gorge. The modern observer can discover a deep and meditative pleasure being around something so old, a great geological wonder that serves as a touchstone for our own origins. Such petrified nature teaches us where we've come as a species. Older people teach us where we've come as a family or a society.

For the gerontologist who studies human aging, a comparison with the Grand Canyon would seem limited. After all, people are not rocks or rivers that age without a purpose and without a genetic code to guide them. The process that continues to unfold in the earth's geography is guided only by the laws of physics, is absent of sentiment, and is still relatively young compared to the age of the universe that bore our planet. But we do have something in common with these rocks and rivers: Both people and geography are aged by two fundamental and immutable forces of nature—time and entropy.

This point was recently made to me by Dr. Leonard Hayflick, one of America's most prominent experts on aging. In 1961, Hayflick published a now-classic paper on cellular aging, informing us that contrary to prior belief, our normal cells could undergo only a limited number of divisions. The Hayflick Limit specifies the roughly forty to sixty times that fetal cells will divide before eventual death, guided in part, it is believed, by the successive shortening with each division of an end region of every chromosome known as the *telomere*. The telomere is like a built-in cellular counting mechanism, with its memory remaining intact even in cells thawed out after years in deep freeze.

At eighty-one years of age, Dr. Hayflick has spent nearly his entire career studying aging, starting in an era of scientific research in the 1950s when "it would be committing professional suicide to mention that you were working in the field" of aging.

In this time he has seen every trend and theory of aging come
along, including the growth of the so-called antiaging industry.
But despite the enchanted claims and pursuits of many researchers in search of a new fountain of youth, Hayflick's view
of aging is quite sobering: It is not a disease to be cured, and
curing all of the diseases that kill us will not extend our own
life expectancy much beyond its current limits. Rather, aging
is an inexorable and inescapable property of every living creature.
And on one level it doesn't matter whether we're talking about
a rock, a river, a cabbage, or a king; aging equals change, and
change is measured by time. To reverse the aging of anything,
we would have to reverse time itself.

We would also have to reverse entropy: the tendency of any
organism's or system's energy to become progressively more dis-
ordered and dispersed, resulting in the weakening of its molecular structure. For example, the rushing waters of the Colorado
River shake the crystalline structure of the rocks over which
they run, breaking them apart piece by piece. The gearshaft of
an automobile engine weathers the heat and pressure of motion
until it either shatters or corrodes beyond repair. And similarly
in biological systems, the molecular bonds within our cells are
inherently unstable. Without constant maintenance and repair,
they eventually fail. As Hayflick writes, "Consequently, the random downward spiral of molecular disorder gradually exceeds
repair or turnover capability and this results in changes in the
cell, tissue, and organ levels that we call aging."

All subtheories of biological aging—and there are many—
stem from this basic principle. The "wear-and-tear" hypothesis,
for example, describes the increasing damage to our cells wrought

gradually and somewhat randomly over time by accumulating antioxidants and toxins, mutations in our DNA, and clumping of sugars and proteins that gums up the functions of cells and tissues. This process of cellular aging, called *senescence*, happens to humans (and many other species as well) once we have reached reproductive maturity. And why does aging begin in earnest then? Humans simply could not exist if we couldn't get to the point where we produced offspring. But once that's accomplished, there is no evolutionary advantage to survival.

Old age, then, is less a product *of* nature and more of a human achievement wrestled *from* nature. Biblical patriarchs aside, the life expectancy for the vast majority of our ancestors was about twenty-five years. We hit close to fifty years by 1900, and then the spectacular medical discoveries of vaccines and antibiotics in the last century enabled most of us to live into our seventies and beyond. And according to the 2000 census, the one-hundred-year-olds are the single fastest growing age group in America. And yet despite these statistics, most of the current resources being put into the science of aging are directed less toward understanding aging or extending our lives and more toward finding ways to make us *look* younger.

The ongoing obsession with finding at least some part of the fountain of youth has an honest origin in our own perceptions of aging. Starting around the age of thirty-five, the face becomes the great oracle of aging. If you look at a series of photographs of someone as he ages, you will see the slow accumulation of distinctive changes in appearance. Below the surface of the skin, a protein matrix of collagen and elastin that gives skin its elasticity begins to break down, as does a thin cushion of fat that supported the once-smooth-and-supple integument above. As a result, the skin begins to stretch, sag, and wrinkle. Small blood vessels weaken and cause the skin to become paler and more easily bruised. And years of sun exposure give the skin a leathery appearance and add dark spots, shaggy growths, moles, red spots, and scabby lesions.

Similar processes of breakdown are happening in every tissue in the body. But even though stiff, aching joints and loss of hair and posture may be both nuisances and affronts to our vanity, Hayflick points out, they are not life threatening. Loss of function in a kidney, liver, or brain due to aging, however, may be catastrophic. Is there a solution? Can we simply treat aging like we treat an infection? There are certainly no shortages of products—lotions, vitamins, supplements, and hormones—that promise to rejuvenate the body and make us physiologically younger. And some researchers have claimed that in the future we will use stem cells or gene therapy to extend life years or even centuries longer.

In response to these suggestions, Hayflick emphasizes that we have not discovered any genes that determine longevity, and so there is no possible gene therapy that could slow aging. Genes do, however, determine the relative integrity of our bodies as well as our individual vulnerabilities to certain diseases as we age. But there is a key difference here between the disease states that increase in frequency with age and the normal but inexorable breakdowns in cellular and tissue integrity that define the aging process. Unlike cancer and heart disease, which can be treated and ultimately cured, aging is not a disease, and thus it cannot be cured. "As of today," Hayflick told me, "we know of no intervention whatsoever that would interfere with the fundamental processes of aging, nor do I think that is going to come about in the future." Exercise, a well-balanced diet, and good hygiene can improve and prop up our biological dwelling places, but age will still come.

But is there any harm in wanting to do better? Hayflick likened the process to trying to extend the life of an automobile. You can repair damage and replace parts, but beyond a certain point the vehicle looks and runs like new only if you've done a complete overhaul. "But that is exactly what you can't do with biological materials," Hayflick reasoned, "and even if you could, would you want to replace your brain? And then would you be yourself?"

Changes in the brain are, in fact, the most demoralizing aspects of aging. In an 1816 letter to John Adams, Thomas Jefferson captured the sentiment well: "Bodily decay is gloomy in prospect, but of all human contemplations the most abhorrent is body without mind." Alzheimer's disease is at epidemic proportions around the world and growing by the day. We have discovered how to bring more and more people to the very frontiers of the lifespan, but at the cost of rates of dementia that exceed 50 percent by age eighty-five. Most youthful projections cast this as the dismal and inevitable reality of aging. And these fears drive an entire movement that seeks to do what Hayflick says can't be done: actually reverse aging.

One of most widely known of these "prolongevists," as they are called, is Aubrey de Grey, a brilliant British computer scientist and self-taught expert on aging who has taken as his life's mission finding a cure to aging. Many like Hayflick dismiss de Grey as a modern-day Don Quixote tilting at the immutable windmills of aging, but his unabashed confidence and omnipresent argumentativeness in the field of aging—not to mention his hippielike appearance, complete with long beard and ponytail—have made him hard to ignore. In his audaciously titled book *Ending Aging*, de Grey approaches aging solely as something that "is really bad for us, however much we would like to forget the fact." Because, in his view, aging is at the root of all undesirable bodily change and disease, it must be combated and eventually defeated. To this end, he has identified seven fundamental causes of aging that he believes can be conquered with sufficient attention and money.

For de Grey, however, the goal is not simply to live longer but to live better. For it would do no good to prolong life indefinitely if we continued to decline, much like the rare but immortal Struldbruggs in Jonathan Swift's novel *Gulliver's Travels*. "Happy Nation where every Child hath at least a Chance for being immortal!" exclaims the protagonist Lemuel Gulliver on hearing of such "excellent Struldbruggs, who born exempt from that universal Calamity of human Nature, have their Minds free and disengaged, without the Weight and Depression of Spirits caused by the continual Apprehension of Death." Such fantasy is dashed in this political satire when Gulliver learns the true fate of these poor creatures, who still live but continue to age into completely morose and decrepit societal outcasts.

Prominent gerontologists argue that de Grey's intent, while understandable, is simply not possible. Still others go even further and argue that de Grey is misguided. Such a radical extension of life would produce a dystopia in which generation after generation would coexist in unimaginable struggles for resources, status, and rank. Grandparents, great-grandparents, and great-great-grandparents ad infinitum would be indistinguishable in age from one another once each member reached a common point of designated agelessness. With a thousand-year lifespan, for example, cherished notions of family, monogamy ("'til death due us part" for nine hundred years?), family, inheritance, and government would be irreparably disrupted. Imagine an immortal Hitler or Stalin!

De Grey and others counter that any such changes in the lifespan would likely be gradual enough to allow society to adjust—just as it has over the last century as thirty years have been added (plus, there could be immortal Einsteins or Mother Teresas!). But ethicist Daniel Callahan is not convinced, arguing that "nature knew what it was doing when it arranged, through natural selection, to have all of us get old and die." Diane Schaub echoes this sentiment: "Senescence escorts us, more or less gracefully, off the stage," she asserts, "making room for fresh generations."

This entire debate reduces the questions of age to a Manichean struggle between death and immortality. Such a dichotomy is a one-way street under which everything we believe about the meaning of aging flows from inescapable biological facts. Either we accept aging as an inevitable and immutable fact, or we abhor it as a tragic and wholly unnecessary state of affairs. Either way we lose ourselves in the picture, forgetting that regardless of whether we live to be one hundred or one thousand, we still have a great deal to say about what will happen in the time of oldness, a time of potential human creativity in which, according to gerontologist Thomas Cole, "the experience and cultural representation of human aging help to constitute its reality."

This point illustrates where the *people* of aging transcend the *process*. The Hayflick Limit tells us that we are biologically finite, but there is no comparable Hayflick Limit to meaning in late life—that is the lesson from the people.

✖✖✖

An astounding discovery in 2007 by an Inuit hunting party along the northern Alaskan coast resulted in the crowning of the Bowhead whale as the oldest living mammal. Imbedded in the blubber of this leviathan the hunters found the metal tip of a harpoon dating back to the early 1880s. Not only did the young whale survive the initial wounding, but it also managed to escape and live another 120 years! This story reminded me of my former patient Eugene, a 102-year-old World War I veteran who once showed me a small bump above his eyelid that harbored a piece of shrapnel from the Battle of Vittorio Veneto in 1918. Though the Austro-Hungarian troops with whom he served lost this decisive battle, he survived to tell (and show!) the tale for another 85 years.

Both of these survivors, man and whale, illustrate important findings from research into the oldest old human beings. Through a combination of genetics and lifestyle, some individuals are able to either avoid or survive the age-associated medical problems that end most lives, shrugging them off like the whale did the ancient piece of harpoon. In fact, many nonagenarians and centenarians are often healthier and more active than their slightly younger counterparts and have mortality rates after the age of ninety-seven that are actually lower than expected. According to a hypothesis by gerontologist James Fries, disease and disability tend to be compressed into a much later and shorter period of time for those living toward the frontier of the age span, up to and beyond one hundred.

Studies of centenarians have yet to identify any genes that bring longevity (and probably never will, according to Hayflick and others), but they have elucidated several common lifestyle characteristics. Centenarians, on average, have delayed onset of most diseases, especially the main killers—heart disease, stroke, and cancer. They are rarely obese, tend not to smoke or drink alcohol to excess, and often have similarly old siblings (There are, of course, outliers like Frenchwoman Madame Jeane Calment, the oldest recorded living human being, who died in 1997 at the age of 122. She reportedly smoked and drank a glass of port twice a day up until the age of 117!). And centenarian women often had their children after the age of 35 or 40, perhaps an indication of the hardiness of their reproductive systems.

We also see that these older minds, when intact, share several common features. Compared to their younger peers, centenarians cope better with stress, tend to be more confident and independent, are generally less anxious and depressed, and have increased levels of life satisfaction, even when their functional limitations are greater. In addition, research with centenarians has found much lower than expected rates of dementia—roughly in the range of 15 to 30 percent. There may be several reasons for this, including more connections between neurons and less genetic susceptibility to Alzheimer's disease. Whatever the factors may be, they cast a ray of light along the frontier.

Despite these findings, clinicians often assign mythic status to their oldest patients and try not to intervene too much when problems arise. I remember being asked to treat a 106-year-old woman who was wheeling up and down the hallway of the nursing home and banging her cane on other residents' doors. My initial treatment plan of "do nothing and let the woman alone" lasted about one week until staff demanded that I intervene more effectively. I was squeamish, worried that my pharmacologic hand might wield the harpoon that dealt the final blow to this majestic life. I pretended she was a mere 90 years old and started her on a low-dose antipsychotic, to good effect. Her 84-year-old son appeared the next week to thank me. "She's happier, and so am I!" he exclaimed. The frontiers of aging had truly fallen, I concluded.

When it comes to the question of what old age means, I often turn to my patients for answers. As psychiatrist George Vaillant remarks, "Old age is like a minefield; if you see footprints leading to the other side, step in them." Is it possible, I wonder, for the aged to distill the lessons of extreme old age into a formula that would guide all of us into this new terrain? After all, the eighty-five-year-olds and older are the fastest-growing demographic group in the county now, and we are all headed that way. But the answers from my patients are often strikingly mundane: "I stopped counting my age years ago," teased one centenarian, whereas another insisted that she didn't feel a day over eighty. Their answers are not definitive, but that is the point. Hope is a viable response, among many, to old age.

But at the age of forty-five, I can reasonably be asked whether my thoughts are just the starry-eyed views of a young man. Am I like Aubrey de Grey but in another cloak (or beard), wanting to project a different and more hopeful view of aging based simply on my own fear of death? Even though this particular question of aging is personal to me, we all know with absolute certainly that we will age, and the vast majority of us will reach old age. And our experience of aging will be influenced by how we imagine it to be. "Just take me out and shoot me before I ever end up in a nursing home," instructs a middle-aged friend, imagining his decrepit body being cast into the bowels of a stinking nursing home before death. And yet I work in a nursing home day in and day out, and I see how life goes on and even flourishes. Under the right circumstances, the imagined grim reaper of old age can seem more like an angel.

In an unexpected encounter at a caregiver's conference, I once had the opportunity to pose this question of age to an older woman who in her day had been an icon of beauty: actress Julie Newmar. In her career, Newmar was a goddess who embodied the charms of youth: as a dancer and singer on Broadway, as a movie star in such iconic movies as *Seven Brides for Seven Brothers*, and as the sultry Catwoman in the *Batman* series of the 1960s. At one point the movie studio insured her legs for $1 million. I expected that aging would be tough for Newmar, especially because a neurological disorder has made it nearly impossible for her to walk, let alone dance. And yet at seventy-six she is an active, articulate, and deeply spiritual woman who feels as vital as ever, with her writing and countless other activities. She was direct with me on what a book on aging would look like: "The pages would be blank," she insisted, because it would be up to each one of us to fill in our own meaning. This reminded me of Cole's view of aging as a mystery that requires meaning rather than a problem that requires solution: "Human freedom and vitality lie in choosing to live well within these limits" of aging, he suggests, "even as we struggle against them."

When I interviewed Hayflick, I expected to hear about his own experience of aging, but he didn't feel that much had changed for him. Instead, he focused on the impressive effects of aging—most of them negative—on his 104-year-old mother, who at the time of our interview was living on her own in Philadelphia, still relatively cognitively intact, but unable to walk because of the severe effects of arthritis on her knee joints. I asked him whether there was the possibility for improvement. Hayflick appreciated all of the efforts to make late life more tolerable, but he was still pessimistic. "For example, I don't think anyone would operate on her knees," he lamented, "but that keeps her so confined to this one room, and her life is four walls." Hayflick also asserted that she could benefit from an attitude adjustment: "She has been led to believe that a nursing home is a terrible place to be. But she cannot be convinced [otherwise]—she insists on staying in that apartment and dying there." And Hayflick was troubled by doctors who were sometimes too negative and fatalistic to believe that anything could be done for their oldest patients.

I have worked with many patients like his mother. They have severe physical limitations and multiple ailments that sometimes evade our most intensive and compassionate efforts to help. More devastating is the loss of hope engendered by these conditions. And it is not surprising to me that Hayflick could unravel the secrets of the aging cell but struggled mightily with the secrets of an aging mother. Understanding the process of aging does not always help in understanding the people. Questions about how we grow old remain.

Long Time Dead?

No one knows what age will bring. We may plot and plan for years to ensure the best old age possible, but circumstances and fate may dictate otherwise. Pity the person who spends countless hours exercising, eating right, and engaging in any of the imagined saviors of time and age and then prematurely drops dead. And then consider the robust and happy ninety-five-year-old woman I once saw in my office who never exercised and always ate the greasiest piece of meat on the plate with all the trimmings. These anecdotes represent the extremes, of course, and certainly do not denigrate the many tried-and-true aspects of a healthy lifestyle that can increase positive outcomes for aging. But we cannot escape the uncertainly of it all.

When young, we often try to cope with this uncertainty by imagining a future in which happiness will reign only if we remain free of pain, terrible illness, severe infirmity, disfigurement, or devastating personal losses. The inverse of this image is that old age will be quite miserable if any of these factors arise. Such myopic perspectives prove depressing and lead us to put old age out of our minds or to avoid too much exposure to old people.

This avoidance can go only so far, however, and sooner or later we face our greatest fears of aging in one way or another, sometimes prematurely as a caregiver for a loved one. In that role even more uncertainty arrives as we are forced to weigh the myriad complex and confusing issues of how to deal with the underbelly of old age. Leonardo, Rosa, and Alberto taught me this well.

❊❊❊

Leonardo's mother, Rosa, lay spread out on the bed like the Cuba of her birth. In the folds of the sheets that traced the contours of her body he imagined the mountains of the Sierra Maestra, rising then falling within the cotton-spun landscape and splaying down to the three harbors of Havana. Her rational mind, like her country, had sent its most precious memories into exile on a distant shore. Despite his deepest efforts, Leonardo couldn't find her. And yet this woman was the guardian angel who had spirited him out of Cuba as a child. When he watched her sleep, he would often conjure the indelible image of their journey to freedom together, with his mother holding his hand tightly as they emerged from a plane into the brilliant Miami sun, the warm wind lifting up the billowing folds of her shawl like wings.

Leonardo would do anything for his mother, but he could neither understand nor accept the transformation that had unfolded over the previous year. A once bright, loving mother had turned cold, confused, and compulsively agitated as she entered her seventy-eighth year. For some time he had tried to ignore or explain away her symptoms, maintaining a delusion of age, like a form of misidentification in which he still saw her as the young woman who had bravely fled Cuba with him because she feared that Castro would send her beloved son off to the Soviet Union for indoctrination. And yet anyone outside of Leonardo saw in Rosa a depressing picture of oldness, full of mental confusion, irritability, anxiety, odors of incontinence, and fits of crying and panic that quickly gave way to screaming, kicking, and flailing at any attempts to redirect or soothe her.

Leonardo's father, Alberto, had no illusions about Rosa's illness, and I witnessed many times his almost violent grief. When he spoke, his entire body seemed to convulse with each phrase, and he vacillated between expressing devastation over the loss of his partner and exaltation over his enduring love for her. His face would twist and spasm as he coughed and choked on his words of concern: "She . . . needs more . . . help . . . now!" A moment later he would calm down, and a glazed look of resignation would release the tension in the muscles around his eyes and mouth. At eighty Alberto had ceased to age well as Rosa's once mild dementia had nose-dived into a state of frenetic pacing, grabbing, and repetitive, nonsensical vocalizations. I tried to explain to both Leonardo and Alberto that such behaviors are commonplace in various forms of dementia, including its most common variant, Alzheimer's disease. But knowledge in this case brought more despair than relief, more questions than answers, and an unquenchable pleading for my expertise.

I always knew when they had arrived for appointments because I could hear Rosa's yelps grow increasingly louder as they approached the door of my office. Alberto was calling me nearly every day for a while—"Doc, I don't know what to do. I don't know what to do. You've got to help me!"—appearing to mimic both his wife's restlessness and her verbal repetition. He was trying hard to maintain some form of vital balance for them, but the days were just too unpredictable. Peaceful hours with his wife alternated with crises: She fell; she hit him; she urinated on the living room carpet. One time he lost control as she was struggling with his attempts to help her in the bathroom. In his rage he cursed at her and shook his fist in her face a bit too close, nearly knocking out a tooth and sending blood spurting from her mouth. Despite her dementia, Rosa was in remarkably good physical shape. In response to their question about how long she might live like this, I once reminded Leonardo and Alberto that the course of Alzheimer's disease, even in its severe stages, was measured in years. "That's a long time dead," Alberto lamented. Leonardo looked away in silent acknowledgment.

I worried about Leonardo's emotional state, but at least he had a supportive wife and a busy job that kept his mind distracted from Rosa much of the day. I worried more about Alberto, seeing that everything he valued in later life seemed to be teetering on a precipice. How much longer could he manage the stress? Old age for him was chaotic, dizzying, and exhausting, what English writer Ronald Blythe has described as "full of death and full of life . . . a tolerable achievement and . . . a disaster." Over time I began to see telltale signs of depression in Alberto; he was persistently sad, tearful, and dejected. He felt useless as a husband, unable to manage the household due to failing interest and concentration. His sleep was constantly interrupted by his wife's awakenings since she had lost all sense of day and night. On some days he would not eat. Eventually, she fell hard, broke her hip, and ended up in the hospital. I thought it would be a respite for Alberto, but he showed up at my office in an even blacker mood. Leonardo was in tow, now gravely concerned about both parents.

As a psychiatrist I am trained to reflexively consider a diagnosis of depression for someone like Alberto. When it's severe enough, treatment for such a depression is optimal when it involves both talk therapy and a course of antidepressant medication. Alberto's generation, however, is sometimes prejudiced against the "talk" of therapy and more interested in a pill that promises a quicker and easier resolution. And I have had many cases of late-life depression that melted away with a little pharmacology, the psychiatric equivalent of a slam dunk. It's incredibly gratifying when that occurs. The power of medications has solidified our view of depression and other forms of mental illness as mere chemical storms in the brain, prompted and whipped up by genes, stress, metabolic derangements, and a host of other factors. The older brain seems particularly vulnerable, especially when it is pockmarked by small areas of dead tissue that choke off the nerve cells that regulate mood.

At the same time, I had to consider a somewhat wider diagnostic picture for Alberto. In a controversial 1995 *Atlantic Monthly* article entitled "Overselling Depression to the Old Folks," psychotherapist Stanley Jacobson argued against the rush to judge all late-life moodiness as a disease. "Old age is reason enough to be depressed if you dwell on it," he asserted, and then broadsided his own colleagues, accusing them of reducing "the struggle of the old to an illness" and contributing "more to the prevalence of depression than to its cure." Despite his polemics, Jacobson was not actually denying the existence of depression in late life, although he did come perilously close. Instead, he was arguing for the restoration of the mind to the clinical picture, reminding us that most of us will inevitably face "the awesome incurability of oldness" and will struggle with that fact. We can't wish aging away and reduce the negative reactions to it to a dysfunctional organ in the head.

With or without a formal diagnosis of depression, however, Alberto clearly needed more from me than a pill. He needed psychotherapy, and he also needed some hope for his wife. He needed to see her somehow get better, even in small measure. Treating him meant treating her, even though she was suffering from an incurable dementia that now was erupting into furious bouts of agitation. Such agitated states are the bane of geriatric psychiatry; they are difficult to understand, notoriously difficult to treat, and the medications that work bring with them a host of new problems and risks. Not too many years ago such patients were simply medicated into oblivion as a chemical form of the chains that had once bound the mentally ill. It's an antiquated approach that I never use, but families still beg me not to turn their loved ones into zombies, preferring screaming over silence, perhaps because screaming indicates that life is still present.

In any event, I now had three patients to treat: a severely agitated wife, a depressed and exhausted husband and caregiver, and an anguished, guilt-ridden son. I spent time counseling

Leonardo individually, talking about his expectations for both parents and his fears of what may yet lie ahead. He was thoughtful and eager to get my advice, but the emotional connections with his failing parents often derailed all logic. He persisted in caring for both with an obsessive-compulsive style that overwhelmed his time and energy, sowed discord with his wife, and yet brought some relief to his crushing grief and guilt. He acted not only out of obligation as a son, but believing in a sacred emotional debt to Rosa that could never be fully repaid.

I started counseling Alberto as well and then added a low dose of an antidepressant, but despite some mild improvement in his mood, the central problem with his wife continued to be an unstoppable source of dejection for him. Rosa had been transferred to the rehabilitation floor of my nursing home and was giving the nurses hell. She refused to get out of bed, and when she was transferred to a wheelchair, she refused to get back into bed. Every effort to care for her was met with fits of panic and screaming. During the day she frequently wandered up and down the hallway in her wheelchair, intruding into other rooms and taking clothes, food, and personal effects from other residents. Even though her walking and balance were terrible following hip surgery, she would sometimes attempt to stand up and stagger out of her wheelchair, one time tumbling onto the nursing station and sending papers, charts, and an overturned vase of flowers crashing to the floor. I was forced to assign an aide to monitor her during waking hours—at the facility's expense—to prevent a catastrophe.

These behaviors went on for week after week without improvement. I took a broad approach and considered a variety of potential disorders that might have been associated with her dementia, such as depression, mania, anxiety and panic, psychosis, and post-traumatic stress. One antipsychotic medication slowed her down a bit but caused excessive drooling, whereas another made her drowsy and even more unsteady on her feet. Two alternative medications from the same class seemed to agitate her more, perhaps because they paradoxically increased the restlessness in her legs, a sure sign of a medication-induced condition called akathisia. A mood stabilizer didn't touch her fury, and several antianxiety medications caused excessive sedation alternating with periods of paradoxical agitation. Two separate antidepressant trials both caused extreme agitation and weight loss; a third one gave her a voracious appetite. I tried every psychopharmacologic trick in my bag, but to no avail. In concert with her internist and neurologist, I ran every possible diagnostic test, hoping that I was missing some hidden organic cause. Nothing revealed itself, and nothing worked. Alberto and Leonardo were initially patient with my attempts at treatment, but with time they lost faith. Eventually, I too lost faith in my ability to understand and heal her condition. This was less an illness and more an act of God, it seemed, and I was stumped.

In such moments of uncertainty, I frequently conjure an idyllic scene. The actual scene took place one evening during a bitterly cold Wisconsin winter when I was accompanying my grandfather on a call to the emergency room. I still see him leaning closely into the faces of several grieving family members, his serious yet kindly expression unwavering as he explained why he was unable to save their beloved older mother, who lay on a gurney several paces away. He held a definitive air of authority in his role as a small-town doctor, swathed as he was in a long white lab coat wrinkled by endless hours of consultations, hospital rounds, and procedures. It was a primal scene in the practice of medicine, the image of the healer at work even as his own limits are exposed. And this scene occurred in a time and place when my grandfather's role as doctor was sacrosanct. Any moments of uncertainty he faced in clinical decisions— and there were plenty—were often absolved by the respect and understanding given him by both patients and families. If he could not heal, then, his patients believed, it was simply beyond the powers of medicine to heal.

My grandfather represented an era of medicine in which doctors held unique esteem in the eyes of society: almost beyond reproach and imbued with an authority and a privilege that drove the doctor-patient relationship. This admiration for doctors has changed significantly since my medical training in the 1980s. The uncertainly of difficult clinical cases is set against a very different backdrop in which the doctor is no longer considered the ultimate authority, where patients sometimes know or think they know more than the doctor about their illnesses by virtue of in-depth Internet research, and where rigid diagnostic and treatment algorithms, managed care criteria, and public scrutiny hold doctors accountable in ways that often demoralize the profession.

Cross the complexity of aging with the plethora of age-associated illnesses and the frustration and hopes of family members, and the geriatric specialist is left with an extremely vexing situation. With Rosa, for example, it was never clear how much of her problem was due to her underlying dementia and how much to a more acute, superimposed illness. How much was due simply to the ravages of age, and how much was due to a potentially reversible illness? This is a central dilemma with all aged individuals and begs the question of how much control we ever have over the inexorable age-associated changes in both mind and body. This uncertainly is frustrating and may drive two opposing attitudes among the aged and their caregivers: a fatalism that accepts the process and is resigned to its inherent suffering and an amalgam of rejection, denial, and simple optimism that refuses to give up and accept the status (call it *stagnant*) quo.

At the same time, many physicians still hold a fantasy of absolute authority, coupled with a desire for the decisionmaking prowess described so cogently in Malcolm Gladwell's book *Blink: The Power of Thinking Without Thinking*. Gladwell holds that many expert decisions are made quickly and intuitively based on a sizing up of the gestalt of a situation. Such decision-making is not the realm of the novice; it requires years of training, experience, and a certain savoir-faire to accomplish. Given the inherent uncertainty of many medical situations, both patient and doctor are rallied by the confidence and *certainty* that such decisionmaking brings. Even some caregivers fall into this fantasy and imagine that they, too, by force of will, can bring about a magical transformation in an afflicted loved one with just the right decision. I have seen countless caregivers wracked with guilt when their efforts prove futile.

However, in two books with different authors but identical titles—*How Doctors Think*—physicians Karen Montgomery and Jerome Groopman both suggest that the rapid "blink" of expert decisionmaking is not always appropriate in medicine. Both authors stress that illness involves "uncertainty, loss of control, and the damage to the sense of self." In the face of this uncertainty, doctors appeal to the science of medicine and the statistical probability of healing to make decisions, but there are pitfalls here. Not every treatment can bring a 100 percent guarantee of success, and having to rely on lesser statistics (such as a 78 percent chance of success or a 5 percent chance of certain unpleasant side effects) can undermine a doctor's confidence in his or her own decisionmaking and can be anxiety provoking to patients and families. At the same time, the uncertainty of medicine allows its practitioners to hide behind numbers or theories rather than face their own inevitable vulnerabilities and even practice failures. Based strictly on the science of late-life illness, the rationale for medical care in the final days of life is tenuous at best. Not surprisingly, a term such as "death with dignity" has become more of a catchphrase in medicine than "life with dignity," as the former term may allow an easy out when there is no certain treatment or certainty of improvement. Ultimately, Montgomery is clear in stating that medicine is a practice, rather than a strict science, in which uncertainty is a normal part of the process and its engagement can bring increased choices, control, and, ultimately, hope.

Groopman, too, argues that uncertainty is an inescapable part of medicine and cannot always be resolved with scientific reasoning. This is a quite disconcerting assertion, implying that even the strictest evidence-based deductive reasoning will not always bail us out. Comparing a doctor to a sleuth, Groopman states that "human biology is not a theft or a murder where all the clues can add up neatly. Rather, in medicine, there is uncertainty that can make action against a presumed culprit misguided." As opposed, then, to the ever-popular Dr. House, like our old literary friend Sherlock Holmes (written, not surprisingly, by *Doctor* Sir Arthur Conan Doyle), who is always able to solve the mysterious illness, real-life doctors are not so easily able to wrap up medical and psychiatric conundrums with a neat bow at the end. We sometimes have no clear answers.

Rosa's case continued to stump me for some time, and so I turned back to the image of my grandfather as the consummate doctor. I realized that it wasn't his absolute knowledge or authority that made the difference in his practice but the two key virtues of persistence and courage, manifested by an unflinching involvement with both patient and family. He tolerated the uncertainty of medicine well, perhaps because he had trained in an era before CT scans, ultrasounds, and even antibiotics were available to seemingly guarantee clear diagnosis and quick healing. The practice of geriatric psychiatry often reminds me of that earlier era, because I face patients with intractable symptoms that cannot be visualized on any scan or diagnosed with any single test. With Rosa it would have been easiest to simply call in hospice and wash my hands of the case, but something in me (call it intuition) resisted. And so I sat down with Alberto and Leonardo and laid out everything we knew—and didn't know—about Rosa's condition, and we discussed all the remaining treatments that we could reasonably consider. This was not a single discussion but a dialogue that took place over many weeks.

Finally, we decided to hospitalize Rosa and try electroconvulsive therapy, or ECT, often referred to somewhat pejoratively as "shock therapy." Despite many misconceptions about ECT, it is actually one of the safest and most effective treatments for severe depression, even in older individuals. A course of ECT typically involves eight to twelve sessions spaced out over several weeks. During each session the individual is briefly anesthetized and paralyzed with medications and then administered an electric shock to the forehead to induce a seizure. We still have no clear idea of how ECT changes brain chemistry to improve depression and other mood disorders, but its effects are impressive. Nevertheless, it's usually a treatment of last resort.

ECT is used even more rarely to treat agitation associated with dementia, but with Rosa I felt we had run out of choices other than massive doses of sedating medications. I feared that the procedure would only exacerbate her underlying memory impairment, but the potential benefits still outweighed the risks. Despite how "long time dead" Rosa appeared to her family, I had to have some hope. Over the course of three weeks Rosa received eight rounds of ECT. Her memory impairment held steady, and she seemed to tolerate ECT well for the first two weeks, but without response. During the third week, however, Rosa's storm began to subside as she grew quieter and less frenetic. Her once fearsome wind became a breeze, and we saw that the treatments were working. Actually, they worked beyond our wildest expectations, and a completely different woman emerged from the hospital. She was generally calm, pleasant, and cooperative. I could actually have a conversation with her. "My wife—she's back!" Alberto exclaimed every time I saw him, and he was back, too. He stopped his antidepressant and dropped out of therapy, telling me, "I don't need it anymore!" Leonardo was equally thrilled, and now Rosa, even in her relatively severe state of cognitive impairment, seemed like a rose. It was as if an exile had returned, changed from the experience and not quite the same person, but good enough. For Leonardo and Alberto, Rosa was home.

Although in retrospect I can claim that the success of the ECT confirmed a clear diagnosis of acute mania in Rosa that was superimposed on her Alzheimer's disease, I realize that this Monday-morning quarterbacking brings no more certainty to the case. After all, every other treatment for mania failed. And so what made the difference in the end? Groopman suggests that "uncertainty sometimes is essential for success." But what does this mean?

There is a lesson here on aging, a moral to the parable of old age that begins with the question of what it means to be old and proceeds, at first, into a realm of great complexity and uncertainty. As a doctor to the aged, I have discovered that I must embrace this uncertainty and hold on tightly, often plunging in up to my elbows and hoping—sometimes against hope— that persistence and faith will prove correct. I have seen, however, that regardless of the outcome, our greatest humanity emerges in the desperate process of caring for someone old and ill. The relationship we establish with our elderly, and with their loved ones and caregivers by extension, ultimately trumps the agony of uncertainty. Over time, uncertainty buys us time, opening up doorways of possibility that reveal as much hopefulness as possible. Absolute certainty may come only with the death of the elder, but that is a fragile certainty lost in its very expression. Old age is not a long death as long as we maintain these vital connections with its inevitable practitioners. For they eventually become us.

Part II
Old Age Rounds

Listen: the sound of your going has a length of its own.

—GARY MIRANDA, "GOING"

Isaac, Erik, and Isak

Beneath the crumbling stone walls and dried-out cisterns of the ancient city of Be'er Sheva, the waters are abundant. Fed by rainfall from the nearby hills of Hebron, the massive aquifer that runs below the bedrock has allowed civilization to flourish in the desert crossroads above. It was here, the Bible tells, that the patriarch Isaac dug wells, raised his family, and sealed an oath with King Abimelech to live in peace with the nearby tribes. This is also where a primal struggle took place between two brothers over who would receive their old father's blessing to become the next head of the family.

According to Genesis 27, by around the age of one hundred Isaac "had grown old" and "the vision of his eyes had dimmed." Knowing that his life was entering its final stage, Isaac asked his son Esau to hunt some game and prepare a tasty meal for him, after which Isaac would bestow his blessing on this son.

Overhearing her husband's instructions and believing their son Jacob to be more worthy of the blessing, Rebecca devised a plan to trick the blind old man. While Esau was out in the fields, she prepared an alternative meal of goat meat for Isaac and dressed Jacob in animal skins so that he could masquerade as his hairier brother. Isaac was initially suspicious, but the ruse worked and Jacob was blessed. Later, Esau appeared with his own tasty meal, and a seemingly bewildered Isaac asked, "Who then is the one who hunted game and brought it to me . . . and I blessed him?" Discovering that he had been tricked by his brother, Esau burned with a murderous fury toward Jacob, who quickly fled Be'er Sheva. In the end it seems an old blind man was fooled and a new generation of conflict was created.

That such drama takes place in the life of a centenarian is nothing new for the Bible, as most of its early characters are wholly geriatric. After all, Noah lived for 950 years; Abraham died "at a good age, old and satisfied" at 175; and his wife, Sarah, gave birth to Isaac well after the age of 70. In the case of Isaac, there is a singular lesson on aging that I take from his story: Sometimes what we perceive only as a weakness conferred by old age may actually conceal or prompt a strength. On the surface, it is a story about a weakened and physically blind old man who could not tell the difference between a ruddy, rough, and hairy son and a smoother, more genteel one. But lying beneath this surface is a man who sees exactly what's going on and who in his deep, abiding love for both sons refuses to expose the wrongdoing of one and the deception of the other. The dimming of one attribute allowed the extension of another, and two seemingly opposite forces—vision and blindness, light and darkness, *Jacob and Esau*—were thus balanced and ultimately reconciled in the life of Isaac. Now the story could continue into the next generation.

As with the actual process of aging, we can easily miss the hidden strengths that guide and balance a person's life. Memory slows down, but knowledge and wisdom increase. The loosening of certain neural connections in the brain may enhance creativity. And the failing of physical strength may prompt the need for greater intimacy and companionship with others. Within each problem lies a solution that enables further development.

I did not learn this lesson originally from my older patients. Nor did I learn it originally from the Bible or from my studies as a psychiatrist. And though I did learn it first from a great thinker who wrote about the human life cycle, it was less the theory and more my encounters with the man behind it— the *old* man behind it, *dimmed* by age—that taught me this lesson. At the time, I was a young nineteen-year-old college student and he was my eighty-two-year-old teacher. His name was Erik Erikson. Like Isaac, Erik was a patriarch, an original force in the field of psychoanalysis and psychology. There are few textbooks in either discipline that do not mention his name and his work as fundamental to an understanding of adult development. In fact, he could accurately be called the father of all life cycle studies.

Getting to know the famous Erik Erikson was a heady experience for a college sophomore at Harvard who still had one foot in the small Wisconsin town of his upbringing. It was the fall of 1984, and during the first week of classes I ran across a flier that advertised a seminar on the human life cycle to be led by Erikson and his wife, Joan, as well as by Professor Diana Eck from the Department of Religion and Dr. Dorothy Austin from the Divinity School. Erikson was returning for a final curtain call at Harvard, where his career in America had begun some fifty years earlier and reached its zenith during the late 1960s. I immediately called the number on the flier to apply for the seminar, and within a few hours I was sitting on a brick stoop in Cambridge being interviewed by Dorothy. I did my best to tell her about myself and explain my interest in the course, but in retrospect I am not certain what I said made any difference. Something just fit, and soon I would meet the master.

Erik Erikson was born in 1902 and grew up in the German city of Karlsruhe, raised by a loving mother who refused to reveal the true identity of his father—a mystery that he would never solve and that would profoundly shape his life and work. He was a Jew who looked more like a Nordic gentile, and he did not feel that he fit in either community. He was not a particularly gifted student. He gravitated toward the arts, studying how to sketch and make woodcuts. But despite his artistic interests, young Erik Homburger (as he was known at the time, taking his stepfather's last name) was moody, directionless, and depressed.

In his early twenties Erikson continued to flounder. He studied art in Munich and spent a significant amount of time traveling throughout Germany and Italy. In 1927, however, his childhood friend Peter Blos invited Erikson to help teach at a

Vienna school for the young children of visiting foreigners being analyzed by Sigmund Freud and his daughter Anna. Through his connection to the small school, Erikson was quickly inducted into the inner circle of the Vienna Psychoanalytic Society. Anna Freud provided direction, a personal analysis, and mothering for Erikson, and he bathed as well in the physical presence of Sigmund Freud himself. Erikson himself recalled the thrill of waiting for a therapy session with Anna and seeing Sigmund Freud emerge from the adjacent office and offer a bow before retrieving his next patient.

In 1930 Erikson was formally introduced to a beautiful twenty-six-year-old Canadian woman named Joan Serson, who was visiting Vienna to study dance. Joan, in contrast to Anna, was a warm and spirited woman who came to eschew the insular psychoanalytic community and its approach, which overemphasized the inner mechanics of the psyche and neglected the outer world of activity and socialization. Not only did Joan give order and stability to Erikson's life, but she also had a profound effect on the direction of his work. He had been schooled by Sigmund and Anna Freud in the strict excavation of memories that formed in childhood and attached themselves to the basic structures of the mind—id, ego, and superego. But in his own work Erikson liberated these memories from both the child and its mental template, showing how they continued to evolve and face unique challenges in the active social world of adolescence and adulthood. In many ways, this shift was all Joan.

She was also a catalyst for their move to America in 1933, where they settled in Boston. Erikson began working as one of the first child psychoanalysts in the city. Throughout the 1930s he built an impressive reputation as both an empathic and successful clinician and a serious thinker about child development. This productive time solidified his identity as a psychoanalyst and as an American, a change symbolized in 1938 by his adoption of a new family name—*Erikson*. The name hearkened back to his Scandinavian roots and proved to be a successful alliteration in his later literary fame

In 1939 Erik was invited to join the faculty of the University of California at Berkeley's Institute of Child Welfare, where he began to work in earnest on his theory of human development. Initially, he looked at how children play, at the shapes, forms, and directions of their toys and games, which are partly influenced by the effects of the developing body on the mind. But in contrast to his psychoanalytic roots, Erik saw no sense in speaking of the role of the unconscious mind forged in childhood without reckoning with the equally important roles of society, culture, and the historical moment.

When the product of his clinical work and research emerged in 1950, *Childhood and Society* had a revolutionary effect on American psychological thinking, which at the time was beginning to demand a greater equality of voices. Here was a psychoanalyst who wrote about childhood development as it took place in middle-class white households across America, on the plains of South Dakota with the Oglala Sioux, and on the Pacific West Coast with the Yurok tribe. In it he coined the term "identity crisis" to describe the process of trying to define self-identity during late adolescence and young adulthood. By the 1960s Erik's work was as apt to be found on the bookshelves of scholars as in the hands of young students protesting the war in Vietnam and trying to define a new identity for America. As his fame was spreading, Erik returned to Harvard to teach an undergraduate course entitled "The Human Life Cycle" (and aptly nicknamed "from womb to tomb" by many students). He had both an unconventional style and a relaxed charisma that resonated with students during the turmoil of the time, and his course quickly became one of the most popular on campus. He was an older man who still commanded the trust of a younger generation seeking to overthrow the establishment. In addition, many of his students were in the throes of their own identity crises and looked to Erikson as a guiding light.

Erikson's career reached its zenith between 1968 and 1973. He won both the Pulitzer Prize and the National Book Award for *Gandhi's Truth*, which traced the life of Mohandas Gandhi set against the template of the life cycle. Considered a cultural icon who graced the cover of *Newsweek*, Erikson was consulted by the academic and political elite. In 1970 he taught his famous course for the last time and retired from Harvard, but awards, honorary degrees, and prestigious lecture invitations poured in. As the 1970s drew to a close, however, Erikson was beginning to slow down considerably, beset by several physical illnesses. During this same time, his theories were subject to greater challenge as the psychopharmacologic revolution brought a paradigm shift to psychiatry and psychoanalytic approaches fell out of favor. "It's all poetry," a professor of mine once declared to me, denigrating Erikson's work as nice sounding but unscientific.

As old age loomed and Erikson faced a number of personally devastating critiques of his work, he was fortunate to have his wife and several close associates to help buffer some of the stress.

And yet ever since leaving Vienna, he had not continued with any form of personal psychotherapy, as he had previously done with Anna Freud. "There is the incredible paradox," his daughter, Sue Bloland, related to me, "in that my father is writing about psychoanalysis in such a brilliant and innovative way, and yet he was rejecting it for himself—and my mother was helping him do it." Daughter-turned-psychoanalyst Bloland believes that it was her parents' very fame that enhanced their desire to hide feelings of inadequacy that had deep roots in their childhoods.

A more profound turning point for Erik and Joan Erikson began in 1984 when they returned to Harvard from California for an encore of their seminar on the life cycle. Within a few years they moved into an intergenerational home in Cambridge with Eck and Austin, hoping that this would provide a satisfactory old age. Despite the creation of a center at Harvard to promote Erikson's work, the regard that his writings had garnered in the preceding thirty years had continued to fade, and outside of professional circles he had become much less known. In fact, other than his name none of my roommates or friends at college knew much else about the man I was about to meet. How I even knew his name was a mystery to me, as I had not read any of his works and had had little exposure to his theories. Yet something gripped my attention when the seminar was advertised, and I was drawn to it for mysterious reasons that now seem fateful.

The life cycle seminar had about twenty participants, mostly drawn from Harvard's School of Education. I was the youngest participant, and Erik was the oldest. It was held late in the day in Sever Hall, an imposing nineteenth-century red-brick-and-blood-mortared building in Harvard Yard that looks itself like a giant brick, adorned with two symmetrical round bays that extend the height of its four stories. We met in one of the ground floor bays, sitting around a long wooden table with the Eriksons at the head.

On the first day of the seminar I arrived with nervous anticipation to meet Erik and Joan. As I entered the room, Erikson stood out immediately, with a burning bush of white hair and a faint frosty mustache. His face was a melding of Semitic and Nordic physiognomies, with a beautifully carved nose and cheeks whose skin revealed the bony prominence of age. His tall frame was somewhat gaunt and slightly stooped but magisterial in its oldness. He was a cross between Moses and Thor, and I expected him to be wearing a white priestly robe and bearing in his hand a giant hammer with radiating bolts of lightning. Instead, he wore the colors of the earth: a brown tweed jacket, a stone-colored shirt, and a bolo tie fastened with a round coin of polished granite. On his feet he wore black socks and brown leather sandals. I greeted him sheepishly, and he shook my hand politely, his demeanor quiet. Joan, in contrast, wore a radiant smile, and she greeted with a burst of energy the students who were slowly ambling into the room. Her shirt, shawl, and long skirt matched the earthiness of her husband's clothes but with richer colors and thicker textures, and she was adorned with a stone-beaded necklace.

There was a celebratory mood to the seminar, a feeling of homecoming for the Eriksons. The crisp fall air outside lent a coziness to the group. Each week we explored a different concept from Erikson's work. The discussions were always led by Professor Eck and Dr. Austin, with Erikson appearing to listen intently, nodding along and occasionally offering a few words. My roommates were slightly intrigued but mostly bemused by my hero worship of him, particularly when I told them how excited I was to shake the hand of someone who had shaken hands with Freud. They called him "sandalman" and suggested that I was devoted to him like a young child skipping after the pied piper.

The fundamental theme of the seminar was Erikson's conception of the eight stages of the human life cycle. The idea of staging the life cycle goes back in history at least as far as the riddle posed by the Sphinx in Greek mythology: "What creature goes on four legs in the morning, two legs at noon, and three legs in the evening?" According to the myth, Oedipus solved the riddle because he knew that a man starts off as a crawling baby, then walks upright as an adult, and finally rests on a cane in old age. These three stages gave way to four and then seven as the notion of the rise and fall of human strength and capability across the lifespan was perpetuated by Greek, Roman, and then European writers and philosophers.

Erikson was particularly inspired by Shakespeare, whose protagonist Jaques in *As You Like It* declares,

> *All the world's a stage,*
> *And all the men and women merely players;*
> *They have their exits and their entrances;*
> *And one man in his time plays many parts,*
> *His acts being seven ages.*

Shakespeare goes on to describe each stage from infant to

Last scene of all,
That ends this strange eventful history,
Is second childishness and mere oblivion;
Sans teeth, sans eyes, sans taste, sans every thing.

Unlike Shakespeare's poetic rendering, however, Sigmund Freud was interested less in mere descriptions and more in the whys and hows of each age as it developed during childhood. He believed that successes, failures, and fixations from early childhood stages accounted primarily for the later vicissitudes of personality and that most major psychiatric symptoms had roots in this development. He proposed that symptoms could be understood and, ideally, resolved through psychoanalytic exploration of the mind. Not surprisingly, old age was a conundrum for Freud, a no-man's-land where psychoanalysis initially dared not tread, not because it lacked the means but because "old people are no longer educable." Though he himself was quite productive in his old age, the younger Freud imagined that the "mass of material" in late life would prove too much for the psychic probing of his fledgling science.

Erikson was schooled in this theory but found it insufficient to describe life after childhood and the vital interaction between the inner psychic structures of the mind and the outer influences of the social world—a process he termed the "psychosocial." The heart of Erik's theory lies in this juncture between the mind and the social environment, at once both a struggle and a merging of opposing forces. *Ego-syntonic* forces stoke the sense of self or ego and promote positive growth, whereas *ego-dystonic* forces lead in opposite directions and produce discomfort, withdrawal, or rigid defensiveness.

This theory underlies nearly everything else that Erikson wrote. In each of the eight stages from birth to old age proposed by Erikson, there is a central tension or crisis that emerges and propels development. In Erikson's lexicon, the word "crisis" "does not necessarily connote a threat of catastrophe but rather a turning point, a crucial period of increased vulnerability and registered potential."

The struggles and resolutions in each stage take place in relationships between individuals and across generations and are carried through into successive stages. The endpoint of each stage, ideally, is a tilt toward the ego-syntonic, along with the acquisition of core strengths that form the foundation of successful growth and adaptation. For example, the adolescent who is able to pick and choose among various "confirming ideologies and affirming companions" and commit to several of them as part of his or her identity can develop a strong sense of *fidelity* that will apply throughout life. In young adulthood, where intimacy versus isolation becomes the dominant theme, the acquired strength of fidelity is now applied to a partner and to work, and a new strength—love—is sought. Erikson didn't stop at the individual; he spoke of how our acquired strengths and weaknesses interact with societal values and historical trends.

At the time of the seminar, Erik fell chronologically into the eighth stage, which centers on the task of developing and maintaining a sense of *integrity* with respect to body, mind, and social network in the face of age-associated pressures and losses. In practical terms, this is a person who can examine her present circumstances and review past experiences and have a sense of completeness, understanding, and meaning. In late life "meaning" refers to both an intellectual and an emotional sense of rightness, harmony, and purpose. It may also represent a transcendent, ineffable mental sensation of connection with a larger entity, such as can be found in nature, spirituality, or love. A person may have suffered greatly in life or may still be suffering, grieving, or feeling pain, but he can still find meaning and achieve a broader sense of integrity in day-to-day existence. This is a gift of aging that can be shared across generations.

Despair—"the feeling that the time is now short, too short for the attempt to start another life and to try out alternate roads"—is the opposing ego-dystonic force in Erikson's eighth stage. Such despair may represent many dystonic forces—mistrust of caregivers, shame over a declining and dysfunctional body, an inability to be industrious, lost roles or identities, isolation from loved ones, and stagnation in daily activities—that have collapsed into one and given rise to an overall feeling of disgust with life. Although cultivating a sense of integrity seems to be the only ideal pursuit in later life, Erikson's framework is more supportive of a balance between syntonic and dystonic forces. This does not mean that a little despair is necessarily good, only that an unbridled sense of integrity without some realization of the limited horizon ahead can be problematic. The achieved balance in perspective— a recognition and tolerance of competing life forces and of the reality of death—is what Erikson aptly labeled "wisdom."

At the time of the seminar I imagined that Erikson embodied the eighth stage. His achievements were monumental, and he seemed to be a fount of wisdom and reflection. I now realize that my nineteen-year-old eyes were unable to see the reality of the situation. Erik was attentive but quiet during the seminars, occasionally adding a comment in his heavily German-accented English, along with a small gesture of his hand or a mischievous smile. Because he was revered by the participants, such responses sufficed as meaningful signs from the master. In reality, he offered little more than his presence, and Joan spoke with enough energy and expression for both of them.

One day at a small reception for the seminar, I approached Erikson to discuss the project I was working on—a replication of his 1930s study on children's play constructions. I caught his attention for about ten seconds until he waved me off, simply stating, "I am trying to eat a cookie." Still too starstruck to be angry, I felt deeply embarrassed for bothering him. My roommates howled at the scene when I recounted it later that night, suggesting that such was the fate of anyone trying to chase a guru. I laughed along with them, hoping to dissolve my own confusion and lack of self-esteem in their rather pessimistic assessment. To this day they occasionally remind me of the "cookie scene" as a hard-learned lesson in hero worship.

As I think back on the seminar from the perspective of a well-seasoned geriatric psychiatrist, however, I now realize quite clearly that Erikson was suffering from early-stage dementia—most likely Alzheimer's disease. The symptoms of this dementia accounted in part for his quiet and apathetic demeanor, his inability to make significant verbal contributions to the seminar, his distance, and even his unwillingness to engage in conversation during the cookie scene. In my clinical work I am similarly waved away multiple times a day by patients who are simply too tired, confused, or impatient to speak to me. Indeed, in a biography of Erikson entitled *Identity's Architect*, Lawrence Friedman recounts how by the early 1980s Erikson's writing projects were "erratic" and required "more energy and perseverance than he could summon."

Fittingly, then, in a revised edition of one of Erikson's last works, *The Life Cycle Completed*, a section written largely by Joan Erikson proposes a *ninth* stage to the life cycle, representing individuals in their eighties and nineties beset by the overwhelming demands and difficulties of everyday life. Much of the description of the ninth stage is quite gloomy as it depicts the unraveling of the life cycle due to bodily decline and the loss of autonomy, self-esteem, confidence, and, ultimately, hope itself, casting despair as the dominant force. She writes that "there is much sorrow to cope with plus a clear announcement that death's door is open and not so far away." This perspective depicts our greatest fears of aging, a projection of how miserable life must be without all of the capabilities we cherish in earlier stages.

The theory of the ninth stage, however, is not well developed and seems to reflect Joan Erikson's struggle with aging more than her husband's own thinking. It may also represent the loss of the attention and adulation that was critical to the Eriksons' identities. For Erikson, however, the loss of memory likely brought with it loss of insight and a loosening of his attachments to lifelong concerns, including a need for affirmation from others. Disappointments from unachieved goals that he might have felt late in his career succumbed to the creeping shadows of dementia. His aches and pains in the final years, like his joys, were those of any other individual, famous or not. It is ironic how dementia steals away personal identity just as it finally liberates the mind from traumatic memories and neurotic concerns.

For Joan Erikson, however, the clarity of her mind until her final days allowed her to care for her husband and promote the vestiges of his fame. It also brought the physical and mental burdens of caregiving and, in the words of their daughter, the "dread of being abandoned by the world should it become known that her link with greatness was no longer viable." But to the outside world, Joan Erikson was unfailingly bright and stalwart, and she seemed the embodiment of integrity.

Thus, Erikson's situation in 1984 contained a clear dilemma. On the one hand, he was an accomplished man who had achieved substantial fame and accolades in his lifetime. Though he was failing physically, he could still interact in socially meaningful ways, and he had the support of his wife and many others. On the other hand, he was suffering from cognitive impairment that made it impossible for him to participate verbally and intellectually at the high level of discourse and writing to which he had been accustomed. According to his daughter, however, no one knows if he ever received any formal medical or psychiatric work-up for these symptoms.

Joan Erikson did her best to prop up her husband and act as if he were his old self, and those who didn't know him well but were awed by his presence—as I was—didn't fully appreciate the difference. At worst, others might have chalked up his quiet demeanor to old age. "Mother did everything possible to sustain this deception," Bloland writes, describing how her mother "publicly denied Dad's intellectual decline, celebrating—and often exaggerating—every sign on his part that he understood what visitors said to him." In fact, in her preface to the revised edition of *The Life Cycle Completed*, Joan Erikson continues to project this façade years after her husband's death: "When Erik was ninety-one . . . following hip surgery, he became withdrawn, and he serenely retired. He was neither depressed nor bewildered but remained consistently observing and quietly appreciative of his caretakers. We should all be so wise, gracious, and accepting of old age when it comes our way." Although these words are poetic and comforting, such a failure to acknowledge the sad reality of dementia, in which individuals are truly bewildered and often depressed, may prompt a clash of expectations among caregivers and lead to undertreatment of legitimate illness. This unbalanced perspective limits our ability to understand the truth about aging and then educate others, particularly young people, about what is real.

Today, an individual with Erikson's symptoms would get complete physical, neurologic, and psychiatric evaluations that included a brain scan, cardiograms, blood work, and neuro-psychological testing, all designed to discover the cause of the cognitive impairment and make a reasonable diagnosis. This information would guide appropriate care, which would include therapeutic activities geared for the afflicted individual's level of ability and medications to enhance cognition or improve symptoms of apathy, depression, anxiety, or agitation. Doctors did less and had less to offer in 1984, but even so, an eighty-two-year-old man with mild dementia who couldn't conduct a seminar would not, perhaps, have been put in the position to try. But in this case the man was Erik Erikson, and it was both ironic and tragic that the creator of the theory of the life cycle failed to live out his own theory. For how is integrity possible without the ability to remember, appreciate, and articulate the scope of a life?

A lesson from Isaac's old age might be informative here. If we cast Jacob and Esau as respective ego-syntonic and dystonic elements in their father's life, Isaac was able to "see" both while simultaneously elevating one over the other. And consider Isaac's blessing of Jacob: "See, the fragrance of my son is like the fragrance of a field God has blessed. And may God give you of the dew of the heavens and of the fatness of the earth. . . . Peoples will serve you, and regimes will prostrate themselves to you; be a lord to your kinsmen. . . . Cursed be those who curse you, and blessed be they who bless you." If we translate this blessing into a wish for a fruitful life cycle, we might say, "Your presence is special. May you receive what you need in life. May you grow to be your own person. May others find benefit in relations with you (or loss in rejection of you)." And in old age, we might affirm, "May your presence still be meaningful to others. May you receive the care you need. May you still retain some strengths. May you benefit from mutual interactions."

And each component of the blessing was true for Erikson regardless of his mental decline. His presence was magnificent, he received an abundance of care from his wife and others, he still retained the ability to experience life and interact in meaningful ways with others, and these relations brought great blessings to those who spent time with him. His old age showed me how to extend the promises of the eighth stage into the seeming despair of the ninth stage for the oldest, frailest, and most debilitated of our elderly, with whom I now work on a daily basis.

Integrity without the benefit of memory is lived in the moment; it is appreciated through the absence of pain and fear, through the mutuality of affection and social recognition, and through the retained strengths of sensory stimulation, laughter, and creativity. My most enduring images from the seminar are just such moments: a birthday party we had for Erikson during which he joyfully kidded with us, playfully balancing a bouquet of flowers on his head; the Eriksons walking hand in hand across Harvard Yard as they departed from each seminar. These moments, when regarded in all their glory, can serve as a powerful counterpoint to the prevailing view of despair at life's end. They represent the triumph of Jacob over Esau, a view to the heavens rather than to the hunt.

And whether we regard Isaac as an actual historical figure or a fictional character, there is no denying that this tale of a father and his sons sits at the cornerstone of three great faiths. Its lessons have shaped how Western civilization defines morality, elevating the spiritual strength of Jacob over the physical prowess of Esau. Erikson's notion of the life cycle also shows how the story of one life plays a role within the culture and history of many others. We cannot measure a life simply from the vantage point of the nursery or the schoolyard, and the shapes of our lives express more than our genetic endowment or the circumstances of our immediate family circle. The true measure of a life must take into account our place in society, in history, and among the generations.

Within the scope of our seminar, it would have been difficult to study an entire life in such depth. Instead, Erikson used Ingmar Bergman's 1957 film *Wild Strawberries* to demonstrate the life cycle, starting from old age and moving back in time. Beginning in the 1960s, Erikson frequently screened *Wild Strawberries* because "I found in this screenplay an incomparable representation of the wholeness of the human life cycle—stage by stage and generation by generation." Midway through the course, then, we joined the Eriksons for an unforgettable movie night.

The basic plot of *Wild Strawberries* revolves around a daylong journey undertaken by a distinguished seventy-six-year-old Swedish doctor named Isak Borg. He travels by car from Stockholm to Lund, where he is to receive an honorary university degree. In the opening scene, Isak is sitting at his desk the night before the trip and reflecting on his current station in life: "I have found myself rather alone in my old age. This is not a regret but a statement of fact. All I ask of life is to be left alone and to have the opportunity to devote myself to the few things which continue to interest me, however superficial they may be." This strong dystonic element of isolation thus begins the story, and we learn that it runs throughout the course of Isak's life.

The next morning Isak and his daughter-in-law Marianne set out, and the trip is laden with highly symbolic encounters, stops, recollections, and dreams that all serve to recall and reconstruct events from his life. For instance, the first stop is at a wooded summer home along the shore, where he wanders into a wild strawberry patch and daydreams about his cousin Sara, whom he loved and had once hoped to marry. He then encounters a young woman and her two male suitors who need a ride, and their presence serves as a constant reminder of his own early years. The group picks up an angry, arguing couple who are perhaps reminiscent of Isak's own failed marriage. He then visits his cold and critical old mother, in whom we see the genesis of Isak's own isolative and moralistic character. He dreams about being interrogated during a medical school examination, and he is flunked by the professor for demonstrating "indifference, selfishness, lack of consideration." It is a damning critique of Isak's life, pronounced in the dream just before he is led out into the forest, where he witnesses his wife having an affair.

As Isak and Marianne pull into Lund, we find that the events of the day and his interactions with his daughter-in-law, who reveals that she is pregnant with his grandchild, have transformed him. Even in his old age he now seems to have a deeper understanding of both the successes and failures in his life, and he is more emotionally connected to the next generation.

In the final scene of the movie, Isak falls asleep and begins dreaming, finding himself again in the wild strawberry patch with Sara. She takes his hand and leads him to the shoreline, where he sees his parents waving in the distance. He cries out but cannot make himself heard. Nevertheless, he feels at peace. Isak has now completed his journey from old age and impending death back to the first stage and his primal protectors; the cycle has come full circle.

There was an electric feeling in the room as the movie ended, the lights came on, and the group looked to Erikson—as if we were sitting with Isak Borg himself. There was a spirited discussion about the movie, but I do not remember much about Erikson's contributions other than his presence. But we did learn some interesting parallels between Erik and Isak. The movie's idyllic scenes along the Swedish shoreline were certainly a reminder of Erikson's own childhood, when he spent many happy summers at his uncle's house in Denmark only twenty miles across the Oresund waterway from Lund. As an adult, Erikson received the same honorary degree and top hat from the University of Lund as did Isak. And Erikson, like Isak, was now facing the end of his career and the ever-approaching reality of death. But how would his own journey end? Perhaps Isak's tale was an inspiration for Erikson, who had hoped that his own old age would bring similar degrees of honor and revelation. This thought hung over me as the evening drew to a close.

Throughout Isak's daylong journey, the timeline of his life jumps among memories, dreams, and encounters from various stages. One moment he is an old man sitting in an abandoned wild strawberry patch; the next he is a young man again, swooning over the beautiful Sara. Bergman's script echoed Erikson's point that the key elements of each stage of life are embedded in every other, almost like a psychosocial DNA. By the time we reach old age, all the previous lessons of the life cycle become lessons of aging. Nothing is lost from the past, and we carry with us, in one form or another, all of the people, places, and experiences we have encountered.

Perhaps this is what I have found so compelling about Erikson's work. His notion of the life cycle gives a meaningful template to life. It shows us where we've come from and where we are heading. It holds out the possibility for change at any stage, even in the last. Memories can be brought up and reconsidered within the ever-changing context of life. There is the potential for a constant resculpting of identity. We might imagine that aging, like any other stage in life, is fixed in time and form and that our declining anatomy is our destiny. But Erikson's message suggests that the trajectory of a life is more like a tributary of water cascading down the side of a hill and then curling off into the landscape below. At first the tributary follows a cohesive line predictably bent by the angle of the riverbed. But then small lines of water etch through the bedrock, twisting under the influence of unseen pores in the earth until they suddenly open like a flower into the aquifer below.

✺✺✺

More than twenty-five years have passed since the life cycle seminar, and yet I am still inspired by my encounter with Erikson. Out of nostalgia I returned to Harvard Yard in 2009 to retrace my steps. Professor Eck and Dr. Austin had aged a bit, but they were still teaching at Harvard with as much energy and enthusiasm as before, and they greeted me as if hardly a semester had passed since we last met. They both reflected on the last few years with Erikson as he struggled with his failing memory. Dr. Austin described a poignant scene in which Erikson would sometimes sit and read over and over again a page from a small notebook in which he had written the titles of his books. Even as his memory failed, he found ways to reconnect with his past. After I left her office in the basement of Memorial Church, I walked along the brick pathway to Sever Hall and stopped near the bay window of my former classroom. I lost myself in a memory about Erikson.

In 1992, I was working as a medical intern at a small hospital outside Boston when an elderly patient was admitted. It was Erikson. I stood outside his room as he lay quietly in bed, clearly in the final stages of both his physical and cognitive illnesses. There he lay, almost like an infant, unable to communicate and totally dependent on the care of the nursing staff. I had once wondered how his journey would end; now I stood witness. It was painful to be so close to a hero and yet so completely unable to make a personal connection. And yet as I reflected on that moment, I realized that a very deep bond of sorts had been established between two generations of individuals and clinicians— a bond that continues to energize my work. I am reminded of what the Eriksons wrote in their final work together: "If, then, at the end the life cycle turns back on the beginnings, there has remained something in the anatomy even of mature hope . . . without which life could not begin or meaningfully end."

And what was this hope? And for whom? One life ends and passes on, and another generation follows. Aging stands at the juncture between the two, and the enduring connection between the stages of life and all of the forces within are united in a brilliant history. Most of us *will* make it to this point, in one form or another. And we will have the chance to look on ourselves and our loved ones and bestow both a vision and a blessing for the future. This is where the trust of the child can engender the hope of the elder.

Out of blindness, Isaac blessed his son for sustenance, courage, and mutuality—what we would wish for every child. Inured to his own faults, Isak was blessed with a final vision of his life, enabling him to reset his most important family connections—an opportunity that we would wish for every elder. And Erik Erikson himself was blessed by the father of psychoanalysis, Sigmund Freud, who suggested that the role of this once young and uncertain artist would be, simply put, to allow others "to see." Erikson's life was a testament to this blessing. So many years ago he opened my own eyes—and those of countless others—to both aging and the entire life cycle that precedes it in ways that bring great meaning and a deeply felt and abundant sense of hope.

Annabe, Bartleby, and the Doctor Who Flunks Aging

I am a rather young doctor, but the nature of my work brings me into contact with some extraordinary characters, both patients and mentors. Sometimes, no matter how many years I have practiced, I still find myself a student to the life lessons offered by these individuals. Here is one such lesson, which I will relate through the life of a patient named Annabe and through the prism of a literary figure named Bartleby, both of whom capture the essence of a condition that no diagnostic manual has yet classified.

The aged patient doesn't always listen to the doctor. In fact, some patients take pride in their resistance, seeing it as a reflection of their still-present autonomy even as they approach the end of their lives. I saw this recently with my ninety-three-year-old patient Ben. "I am trying to walk *without* my cane," he told me emphatically as he wobbled out the door of my office. The grin on his face was telling as he attempted to stride through the clinic, blissfully unconcerned that the tip of the cane held uselessly behind his back was smacking into nearly every object in its path. I grabbed his arm as he suddenly lurched toward me in the hallway and implored him; "Ben, how about walking *with* your cane, as the doctors have asked?" Ben just smiled at me, pretending not to hear, and meandered out of the clinic. There wasn't much else I could do. I did not agree with Ben, but I did admire his fortitude and positive attitude. Of course, I say this without intending to sanction or romanticize his behavior—or the broken hip that I feared would result.

Unlike Ben, there are older patients whose resistance appears to the doctor to be both negative and life threatening. Such individuals inspire a sense of obligation to help them, but their refusal to cooperate leaves both doctor and caregiver feeling quite helpless. In more extreme cases, these individuals refuse all tests, treatments, and medications, choosing instead to isolate themselves and wither away without clear reason. And herein lies the case in question, perhaps my greatest failed case as a doctor. What I hoped was a straightforward case of late-life depression ended up defying all of my diagnostic wit and pharmacologic sleight of hand.

❈❈❈

I think of a T-square when I think of Annabe, because in every clinical encounter she was lying horizontally on the bed and I was standing vertically at her side. Even when I sat down next to her, the perpendicular positioning of our meeting only reinforced the fact that we were on such different planes. If only the forty-five-year age difference between us had been the degree of an angle, we might have both had a better vantage point for talking. But that, sadly, was elusive. Her doctor had asked me—rather, *begged* me—to see Annabe because for months she had been refusing everything but food: no blood draws, no baths, no touching of her extremities, no trips out of her room, no visitors. Her soft, raspy voice was articulate, and her responses were curt: "Annabe, how about a bath today?" the nurse would ask, and Annabe would reply, "I'd rather not."

Anyone who is a fan of Herman Melville might immediately be reminded of one of his most intriguing short stories, called "Bartleby." This nineteenth-century tale concerns the struggle of a well-meaning but wholly perplexed attorney to deal with his new employee, Bartleby, who works as a scrivener (or copyist) of legal documents. Bartleby is an odd but initially industrious man who will copy documents endlessly but when asked to do anything else simply replies, "I'd prefer not to." The attorney's disbelief and then astonishment at Bartleby's audacious resistance quickly turn to frustration and then confusion over how to handle him.

For me, Annabe *was* Bartleby. Her resistance, like her very presence at our facility, seemed at first to emerge out of nowhere. She had been transferred from a hospital to our rehabilitation floor and then to a long-term unit, pushed along by an unseen force and without the benefit of any human advocate—family, friend, or otherwise. She suffered from a relatively severe post-polio syndrome and was nearly quadriplegic. She was laid out flat like a board, simply garbed in a shabby white nightgown and covered with a sheet up to her neck. Day after day she lay in bed impassively staring at the ceiling, requesting nothing and refusing everything but a few spoonfuls of broth and Jell-O and an occasional swallow of minced chicken that the nurses could coax into her. She denied feeling depressed or suicidal, but her words seemed to betray a deep hopelessness, as she stated that she would rather not have her existence prolonged any more than necessary. A review of her chart revealed several recent aggressive attempts at antidepressant treatment that had all failed. And now she refused further attempts.

Bartleby, like Annabe, eventually refuses all requests, in his case to copy documents, responding to every entreaty from his boss with the same expression: "I would prefer not to." The attorney's anger is tempered by his perplexity at such an individual as Bartleby, and at times he even feels compassion for such a pitiful figure. As the attorney begins to plot ways to rid himself of Bartleby, now an impassive figure who continues to live in the office space without agreeing to perform any work, he questions his own beliefs: "Again I sat ruminating what I should do. Mortified as I was at his behavior, and resolved as I had been to dismiss him when I entered my office, nevertheless I strangely felt something superstitious knocking at my heart, and forbidding me to carry out my purpose, and denouncing me for a villain If I dared to breathe one last bitter word against this forlornest of mankind."

Even as I felt sorry for this bewildered attorney, I fantasized that he and Melville's other literary characters could emerge from the story for a moment to discuss our mutual, parallel circumstances. In my own case, I tried repeatedly to convince

Annabe to eat more food, to accept some physical therapy, to let the nurses bathe her, and to try another antidepressant, but I was always met with the same ninety-degree sigh and terse "rather not." The nurses were growing increasingly frustrated, and the nursing supervisor fearfully envisioned the arrival one day of a long-lost relative or a crusading ombudsman who would sanction the facility and its staff for the insufficient care of this pitiful woman. During one behavioral team meeting I had a mild fit of passion and loudly questioned why we had admitted Annabe in the first place and how we could find another facility for her. Egged on by my fury, the director of nursing demanded that I immediately send Annabe to the psychiatric ward. I knew that I *could* do it—but what would that accomplish for Annabe? It would relieve us of a burden for a few days, at least, but it would have been akin to dumping Annabe on some other un-suspecting party—much like my literary counterpart attempts to do. My passion subsided as my conscience got the better of me, and I slunk away from the meeting resolved to do nothing other than continue my angular reverie at Annabe's bedside each week.

In a like manner, Bartleby's resistance is maddening to the attorney, yet he is unable to resolve any plan of action to re-move the creature from his office. Instead, he moves his entire office and staff elsewhere, leaving Bartleby alone in the empty space. Soon enough, the new tenants arrive at the attorney's doorstep, seeking his guidance on what to do with Bartleby, who now haunts the hallway outside the attorney's previous of-fice. The attorney returns briefly to confront Bartleby, pleading with him to accept some help finding a new job or a home; the attorney even offers to have Bartleby move in with him! But still the same response: "I would prefer not to."

Annabe, like Bartleby, similarly refused every entreaty. "How about a new room?" I asked, "or some fresh air? I will ask a nurse to wheel you out into the garden by the birdcage. Do you like music? We have a wonderful music therapist!" I was getting desperate, but I didn't fold. "How about a different diet? Or a friendly visitor?" I sent in one of our psychologists for a visit, followed by the geriatric psychiatry fellow when that failed, and then an eager medical student, all to no avail. In the next wave, I sent one of our most dedicated volunteers to see Annabe. When that didn't work, I ordered a new antidepressant. "I'd rather not take it," she told me. Finally, I sent in Stuart, our prized "Volunteer of the Year," known for his sense of humor. "Try jokes," I said, "or that Brooklyn routine you do that worked so well with Stanley the misanthrope upstairs." It didn't work, and Stuart was not elegant in his assessment of Annabe. "She's crazy!" he told me, "and whatever you're doing, Doc, it *ain't* working!" I was deflated. I had no good diagnosis, I had not established any doctor-patient rapport, I had achieved absolutely no progress, and I was quickly earning, I feared, the derision of all staff that had to care for Annabe.

I tried to discern some meaning in Annabe's behavior, but I knew almost nothing about her background and had no informants. On the one hand, I knew from my clinical assessment that, even though she seemed depressed, apathetic, and even suicidal at times, she was not demented. On occasion she would explain her reasoning to me, and even though I disagreed, it came from a fully oriented mind and followed a logical line of thought. Her voice was so faint at times, yet it boomed out a consistent set of wishes, and I felt obligated to respect her right to refuse treatment. On the other hand, her depressive and apathetic tone and the way it suffused her attitudes toward accepting care did seem to warp her capacity to make reasonable decisions. The case was poised on the edge of two opposing lines: Leave her alone, or send her to the hospital for electroconvulsive therapy.

I thought about the many reasons that older patients may refuse help. The most obvious explanation is that the individual is so depressed that he or she lacks the motivation, energy, or will to get better. In these cases, resistance to care is sometimes best viewed as indirect life-threatening behavior, a form of suicide. Other individuals simply deny that they have a problem that warrants treatment, perhaps due to ignorance, lack of education, or a condition called anosognosia in which brain damage, usually to the right hemisphere, has robbed them of insight into their deficits. Individuals with personality disorders are also frequent refusers, particularly those with passive-aggressive, depressive, dependent, or obsessive-compulsive traits. Annabe fit some criteria from these various categories, but none of them captured her.

As much as Melville provided some insight into my own reactions, I needed to seek higher counsel. This I found in a thick, prized volume on my bookshelf that had been inscribed to me many years prior when, as a young college student, I had spent some time in the presence of the author, who was not only a famed psychiatrist but also a great Melville scholar—Henry A. Murray. As one of the founding fathers of personality study (a distinction that had even brought him into Freud's study during a visit to Vienna in 1936), Murray saw in Melville some of the richest personality descriptions in all of American literature. In one particular essay Murray had channeled the characters from Bartleby—including Bartleby himself—into a group discussion about the meaning of their lives. I imagined that Murray's Bartleby also gave voice to Annabe as he stated, "Tired of everything, I had resigned myself to—well, a sort of death in life, and then to no life, the last resource of an insulted and unendurable existence. . . . I also derived some hidden pleasure from witnessing the disturbance I produced in the office, seeing to what extent I became the center of attention, and how, one after the other, they adopted my word 'prefer.'"

Was this it? I wondered. Annabe, like Bartleby, was no passive wisp but a lion under a sheet, displaying not the lack of adherence to treatment that we saw but a fortitude "marked by . . . adherence, despite everything, to the principle of self-sovereignty, the last stand of an oppressed ego." If I turned the angle around—now Annabe upright and me horizontal—I began to see a different configuration. This is not to deny the role of psychiatric illness here, and I take Murray's suggestions that Bartleby (and Annabe) could have suffered from a variety of maladies: anger, obsessive-compulsive disorder, regressed behaviors, and the apathy of the institutionalized. Perhaps none of these terms are adequate and a new clinical entity is required: "I will end," Murray declares, "by crediting Mr. Melville with the discovery of the Bartleby complex."

At the end of the story, Bartleby is taken away to a penal institution, where he continues to refuse all requests, even to eat. When the attorney returns for a final visit, he discovers the wasted form of Bartleby lying on the ground huddled next to a wall, his head touching the stones. "He's asleep, ain't he?" questions the cook observing the scene, to which the attorney replies, "With kings and counselors," realizing that the now-mythic Bartleby has passed on. The attorney concludes his tale by relating something he learned about Bartleby several months after his death: He had previously worked as a clerk in the Dead Letter Office. The attorney realizes the tragic journey of both Bartleby and these Dead Letters, consigned to the flames containing perhaps "a bank note sent in swiftest charity—he whom it would relieve nor eats nor hungers any more; pardon for those who died despairing; hope for those who died unhoping. . . . On errands of life, these letters speed to death."

Seized with emotion, the attorney cries out to the reader one of the most famous lines in American literature: "Ah, Bartleby! Ah, humanity!" Critics may debate the meaning of these lines, but as I hold level in my mind the visages of both Bartleby and Annabe, I understand their passionate cry, how they speak to the unfortunate but common fate of so many elderly individuals.

And thus I have tried to understand Annabe by changing the geometry of our relationship, actually upending my own expectations of her behavior. All of us caring for Annabe expected and eventually pleaded for her to act like a patient and obey two key responsibilities of the "sick role" described by sociologist Talcott Parsons: that she have a desire to get well and that she seek out medical assistance. Instead, she expressed the opposite desire and thwarted our very mission to heal her. Not surprisingly, such individuals produce a lot of unwanted conflict with doctors and come to be viewed as "bad" patients.

And so poor Annabe, like Bartleby, did not receive the sustenance intended for her, and she passed away quietly in her bed one morning, without anyone in attendance or even aware of her departure until several hours later. Sometime after her death I was finally able to review some old records on Annabe from the archives of the veterans hospital in which she had spent much time. These few details I learned: Annabe was born in rural Minnesota to a Norwegian minister and his wife, who died in childbirth. She was initially raised by a young couple in the parish, at her father's request, and then later by an aloof stepmother after Annabe's foster mother died suddenly. After high school she became a nurse in the U.S. Navy on the eve of World War II. Although she suffered from a debilitating bout of polio, Annabe recovered sufficiently to be sent to a field hospital in the South Pacific during the height of the war. Here she was traumatized sufficiently by her exposure to dead and dying soldiers and had to be discharged for psychiatric reasons, listed as alcoholism and war fatigue (and later diagnosed as post-traumatic stress disorder, or PTSD). By her early seventies Annabe's drinking had became so severe that she was unable to function and had to be placed in a veterans home with a diagnosis of dementia. Now abstinent by necessity, she slowly recovered her faculties and was discharged to an assisted living facility. Just as she was beginning to live again, she developed a severe postpolio syndrome that robbed her of her ability to walk and later her ability to coordinate her trunk and arm movements. Annabe was passed from one facility to another until she eventually reached our doorstep.

And so there it was, a life of certain emotional deprivation from the very instant of birth, never having a consistent loving parent to meet her needs. This loss was coupled with the shattering experience of tending to dying soldiers who were leaving young children waiting for fathers who would never come home, wives hoping for children who would never be born, and parents dreaming dreams that would remain forever unfulfilled. At certain moments when I think about our attempts to help Annabe, I feel a twinge of the emotional cry expressed at the end of "Bartleby." Her fate was like that of many unfortunate elders: destined to lie in bed alone, debilitated and dependent on the care of strangers, bereft of dignity, and even scorned before death!

At some point Annabe rebelled against this, refusing to accept what life had given her and declaring that perhaps it is better to be scorned than to be ignored or forgotten. Some unconscious siren called out from her stillness, luring all of us into the desired role that had proved so elusive in her life. She died alone but not forgotten and not without concerned attendants, even if that concern was not always so tender. I understand Annabe a little better now and realize the limits of my profession. Sometimes mothers and fathers or their loving surrogates must intervene where doctors cannot. Absent them, we are all in Annabe's position.

Joseph Red Hair

"I cannot compete with a holy man."

This was the solitary thought running through my mind as I sat and listened to my patient. Joseph Red Hair had many identities, some empowering, others expressing great pain and struggle—Korean War vet, PTSD sufferer, recovering alcoholic, and Lakota tribal elder. At sixty-two he was my *youngest* patient, but aged by experiences during combat that, once revealed, were beginning to unravel our work together. On this particular day he told me of his time with a *wichasha wakan*, or Lakota holy man, who had tried to cleanse him of his intense wartime guilt through a sweat lodge ritual. In my own eyes I was feeling somewhat inadequate as his therapist, wondering how I could ever understand and treat Joseph as the holy man did. What words of wisdom, comfort, or healing could I—a child of the 1970s and son of Western culture—give to this man, a child of the

1930s, son of American Indian culture, and descendent of Crazy Horse? Where was the common ground on which to meet, young doctor with older patient?

Joseph Red Hair was a member of the Lakota tribe, also known as the Oglala Sioux, and he had grown up on the Pine Ridge Indian Reservation in the Black Hills of South Dakota. The land of the Lakota was once a vast undisturbed prairie— an "ocean of grass" stretching from Wyoming to Minnesota where buffalo roamed in the tens of millions before being senselessly slaughtered by American settlers and the U.S. Cavalry. Lakota culture revolved around the buffalo, which were hunted for both physical and spiritual sustenance and from which every last piece of flesh, hide, bone, and sinew was put to use for food, shelter, clothing, utensils, and ritual items. Starting in the mid-1800s, the Lakota suffered one devastating blow after another: loss of land; slaughter of the buffalo; disease, war, and massacres brought on by settlers and soldiers; and, ultimately, an education stripped of traditional ways that was forced on Lakota children during the early twentieth century. Joseph's lineage was touched by all of these events: He was a descendent of the great Lakota warrior Crazy Horse; one of his grandfathers had fought at the Battle of the Little Bighorn in 1876, in which Lieutenant Colonel George A. Custer had been killed and the U.S. Seventh Cavalry defeated; and he had lost relatives in the 1890 massacre at Wounded Knee. Joseph was raised in a family stripped of its spiritual basis and crippled by alcoholism. He was saved, he believed, by the powerful and soothing figure of his grandmother, who plucked him from an abusive home and raised him as her own son.

In 1951, at the age of seventeen, Joseph enlisted in the U.S. Army Paratroops, and he soon found himself in ferocious combat on the frozen plains and hills of Korea. His experiences, at least the ones he shared with me, were horrific. He recalled, haltingly during one session, a battle in which an army buddy was blown up in front of him, showering him with brain tissue. He fell into a dissociative stupor afterward, and once he came to his senses, members of his platoon gave him alcohol to soothe him. Alcohol soon became the chosen medication for his intense stress, and he drank heavily. But worse things lay ahead.

In June 1952 Joseph was stationed in Japan as part of the 187th Airborne Division. He and his buddies were out drinking one night when they were recalled to base for what they thought was another drill. Joseph tucked a bottle of I. W. Harper Bourbon Whiskey under his arm and started going through the motions of preparation. Only when live ammunition was being handed out did he realize that his battalion was being sent on an actual mission. Mail call arrived just before Joseph boarded the C-46 troop transport plane, and he learned from a letter that his beloved grandmother had died. He was stung by the news, but he recalls that the pain eased after he took a shot from the whiskey bottle he had in his possession.

Flying into a thunderstorm, the plane climbed and then dropped suddenly, its fuselage shuddering back and forth and sounding like it was coming apart. Joseph was terrified. As he sobered up and grew increasingly grief-stricken over the loss of his grandmother, he became convinced that he would die on the plane, especially after hearing on the radio that another plane had gone down. "I went to a wall in that experience,"

Joseph related to me. "I kinda know when people go insane. I went to a wall where I was experiencing total fear and horror. I prayed my grandmother's prayers, and I did everything I could do in my mind and heart and spirit to take me to a place where I could accept death. I thought about my ancestors in the spirit world, and then all of a sudden I had a sense of peace."

Joseph does not recall the rest of the trip, but on arriving at Koje-do Island off the southern coast of Korea, he and his men were ordered to retake a prison camp that had been commandeered by thousands of Chinese prisoners. According to Joseph, the mission went awry when several of his men were killed during the assault on the camp, perhaps due to friendly fire in the haze of the smoke used as camouflage. Joseph described the deep rage that erupted among the troops, so that "when the Chinese dead were brought out of the compound, people drew their machetes and started cutting heads, arms, and legs off and put gasoline on them and started burning them. And if you've ever smelled burning flesh, it never leaves you." Joseph recalls incongruous feelings of fascination and rage mixed with revulsion, fear, grief, and guilt.

Decades later it was still hard for him to reconcile these actions. "I never thought I would participate in something like that. That's the thing that bothered me for a long time. I came from a peace-loving family. My grandparents were very spiritual people and very gentle, and here I was participating in something that I know now any human being would be driven to that point to act out and to commit those atrocities." It was warfare, he reasoned, and yet the trauma left an indelible mark. In his mind, he descended into a place of evil, inhabited by the Lakota spirit Iya, who is responsible for all other evil beings in the world and who brings only destruction and suffering. According to tribal legend, Iya would disguise himself as an abandoned infant who, once rescued and brought unwittingly into a tribal camp, would swallow it up in one gulp.

In the years following that mission, Joseph sensed the presence of Iya and other spirits in his dreams and visions and in the shadows of his daily life. On some nights he would be visited by a faceless buddy from his platoon who appeared out of the shadows and entreated him: "We've got to talk about this." He struggled with intense guilt and tried, for years, to drown it in alcohol. As a result, his life played out much as the Korean War had, with arduous battles advancing him forward, alternating with retreats in the face of enemy hordes, eventually culminating in a tense truce along an artificial border. For Joseph, the advances were marriage, children, an educational degree, and a stable teaching position, forced back time and time again by endless waves of beer and liquor and furious hordes of slain enemy troops who haunted his memories and visions. Most painful was the fact that when Joseph was visited by these spirits, they appeared to him like his own people, their Asian physiognomy resembling that of American Indians in general and of some of his relatives in particular. He felt unable to conduct the Lakota ceremonies once used by his ancestors to ritually honor the spirits of those they had killed in battle. He was stuck with an uneasy armistice, living both on the reservation and in a large city miles away, seeking wisdom and healing from both a wichasha wakan and a psychiatrist.

When I first began seeing Joseph, I wondered whether he was experiencing transient psychotic symptoms because his "visions" sounded like hallucinations. Yet his spiritual tradition provided a better explanation. In Lakota culture, both dreams and visions hold the key to understanding a person's life and destiny, and they are actively sought and interpreted. According to Lakota teachings, a Lakota spiritual leader once had a vision of Iktomi, a spirit of mischief and teacher of wisdom, who appeared in the form of a spider and wove for him a web in his ceremonial willow hoop. This woven dreamcatcher was Iktomi's gift to the Lakota people to help collect good ideas, dreams, and visions, while letting the bad ones flow through the open center. Many American Indians hang these circular dreamcatchers above their beds, decorated with beads, yarn, and feathers. Joseph's dreamcatcher, I imagined, had collected many good forces in his life, including warm visions of his grandmother and ancestral land, bonds with his children, and the powerful and protective image of a spirit named Standing Buffalo. At the same time, the dreamcatcher was clotted with other forces that couldn't find a way out: gruesome battle scenes, sneering faces of enemy soldiers, alcoholic binges, and infidelities. These inescapable, haunting memories drove Joseph's alcoholism for many years and remained even after he became sober for good. Sitting in my office, I saw a clear case of post-traumatic stress disorder.

PTSD, once referred to as war neurosis or combat fatigue, did not come into prominence as a psychiatric illness until the 1980s, largely driven by the experiences of Vietnam War veterans. The clinical picture of PTSD centers on the intrusive re-experiencing of traumatic memories, often in the form of flashbacks or nightmares, and accompanied by intense fear and physiological arousal. The brain of the PTSD sufferer is stuck in the trauma, unable to separate the memories from the physiological fight-or-flight response that was adaptive during combat but crippling at all other times. Persistent hyperarousal develops as a response to imagined threats and is characterized by insomnia, irritability, angry outbursts, poor concentration, an exaggerated startle response, and hypervigilance. Individuals suffering from PTSD will try to avoid thoughts, feelings, people, and places that trigger these painfully charged memories. This avoidance may evolve into loss of memory for certain aspects of the trauma, decreased interest in activities, detachment from relationships, and loss of hope for the future. PTSD is typically associated with severe depression, anxiety, and substance abuse. Ironically, in severe PTSD the very brain structure that is responsible in the first place for coding the traumatic memories—the hippocampus—is known to shrink over time and impair verbal memory function, perhaps in response to persistently elevated levels of the body's stress hormone cortisol.

When I began seeing Joseph in the mid-1990s, a number of forces were coming together at the same time to change our understanding of late-life PTSD. Veterans Affairs (VA) hospitals were, by necessity, evolving into geriatric facilities treating growing numbers of aging World War II and Korean War veterans. At the same time, veterans who had previously coped with or suppressed underlying PTSD were now appearing with old symptoms triggered by the trauma of age-associated stresses such as retirement, medical illness, or loss of spouses and other loved ones, as well as by many events of the time: the first Persian Gulf war and the growing number of fifty-year anniversaries of World War II events. Many of these veterans had always suffered from PTSD but without a formal diagnosis and thus without treatment. As word got out in the VA system, they arrived in droves, Joseph Red Hair among them.

Like many older veterans with PTSD, Joseph had been treated with both individual and group psychotherapy and was already on an antidepressant when he came to see me. His symptoms were still severe and caused a chaotic life beset by nightmares, depressed and anxious moods, and periods of suicidal thinking. He had been able to maintain a tenuous sobriety, largely due to an inpatient stay at a national treatment center and the strong support of his third wife. I was never quite sure whether he would show up for appointments, because he canceled frequently and was difficult to track down. When he missed an appointment, I could sometimes reach him by phone at his house in the city. Many times he disappeared for weeks on end, traveling either back to Pine Ridge or to some other, unknown place. Even as he began to divulge more of his life history, he resisted my treatment suggestions, asking instead that I wait until he was able to consult the wichasha wakan and revisit the sweat lodge.

As Joseph began to describe more detailed and gruesome memories, he reduced the frequency of his visits, and I started to doubt my effectiveness as a therapist. I tried to limit how much he told me, knowing that his words were triggering an overwhelming flood of emotions. There is a strong nonverbal component to memory that is easily triggered in PTSD. These experiential memories are beyond words and will persist in older individuals despite extensive talk therapy and even in the face of impairments in memory and other mental abilities. Joseph sought relief through traditional Lakota ceremony, in which the holy man sought to restructure Joseph's experiences in the sweat lodge through prayer, chanting, drumming, the burning of sage and cedar, and the interpretation of visions and dreams. The image of a braided Lakota warrior named Standing Buffalo was given to him as a form of guardian angel to guide and strengthen him in his quest.

Over time, I sensed that I was losing Joseph as a patient, and I was sure that the wichasha wakan wasn't faring any better. Joseph didn't seem ready to fully trust either one of us, because his symptoms persisted regardless of the setting, whether in the sweat lodge or on the psychiatrist's couch. His last message to the clinic spoke of his misery but did not betray the fact that I would not see him again: "The patient needs to reschedule the appointment—he's paranoid about coming in today."

Everything I knew about Joseph Red Hair was spoken to me, and yet I understood that, although healing would begin with words, resolution would be found beyond them. There was a primal emotional force sustaining his symptoms, born out of a cauldron of horrific wartime experiences and conflicting emotions that no eighteen-year-old should have to face. His ancestral world had already been shattered, and now his personal one shared the same fate. He had crawled away physically alive from the battlefield, dousing the pain with alcohol, and he had even managed to make a life, but the spirit of Iya—of evil and destruction—was his frequent companion. I suspected that as much as Joseph despised and tried to avoid this force, he also embraced it as a well-deserved punishment, a perpetual act of atonement for his self-described evil actions.

My position with Joseph was not unlike that of many colleagues in geriatric psychiatry who attempt to understand and empathize with individuals of advanced age who suffer from multiple medical problems and often come from vastly different backgrounds. Sometimes these patients are unable to even communicate verbally due to language disturbances (known as aphasia). When patients do not feel understood, or do not sense that there is a shared mission with the doctor, they often retreat—directly by not returning to the doctor or the clinic or indirectly or passively by not following treatment directives. The clinician, in turn, may lose hope in the patient's ability to get better.

The antidote, it seems, is to cultivate a sense of empathy for the patient, to be able to creatively imagine what he or she is thinking and feeling, and to mentally "oscillate from being observer to being participant to being observer." The expression of empathy requires the capacity to listen closely and the ability to respond with physical attentiveness through eye contact, physical demeanor, and voice cadence, all of which indicate some degree of emotional resonance. Empathy also extends beyond the words exchanged between doctor and patient. At the same time, a good doctor must maintain appropriate boundaries without succumbing to his or her own emotional reactions to "feeling" a patient's pain. Unbridled empathy, without boundary, purpose, or true positive regard for the patient, can become manipulative, misleading, and even destructive. It can rob the patient of autonomy.

When working with older patients, including Joseph, I cannot always empathize with experiences or emotions that are foreign to me. How can I know what it is to be ninety-eight? Or to face the death of so many beloved friends and relatives? Can I really imagine what Joseph felt in the heat of battle or after he saw the physical destruction of his buddy? Frankly, most of us do not want to even imagine such experiences and emotions. And when we do, we can wind up feeling depressed, emotionally depleted, even traumatized. Such moments are like comforting a mourner, when words fail us and the best we can do is to simply be present in his or her grief.

In these situations, there is a mutual virtue of hopefulness that is crucial to healing and that goes beyond the spoken words of the doctor-patient relationship. According to Erik Erikson, hope "is the enduring belief in the attainability of fervent wishes, in spite of the dark urges and rages which mark the beginning of existence." It is "both the earliest and the most indispensable virtue inherent in the state of being alive." Hope is a human strength shaped by the mother-infant bond prior to the formation of verbal memories, and it lays the basis for trust in others. When empathy is difficult to conjure, then, we can still share with others the hope that a better state of physical and mental health can be achieved, regardless of the situation. Even with terminally ill patients, the doctor can seek to improve health through reduction of pain, relief of depression, and restoration of personal dignity.

Thinking about Joseph, I realize that the wichasha wakan and I shared this virtue in our work with him. This hopefulness was both a nonverbal sense of communion with him and a more mature, verbally expressed hope—perhaps better termed "optimism"—that he would get better. I could not offer him the burning of sage or the beating of drums in my office, but I could offer my genuine intent to listen to him, to be present for him, and to guide him through the best that Western psychiatry could offer.

Many older individuals who successfully adapt to aging do so by returning to and reinvigorating symbolic pursuits full of meaning and hopefulness that capture the basic trust of early childhood. Others are not so successful, and lacking this hope, they become preoccupied with the immediate gratification of basic needs for food, warmth, bowel and bladder release, physical touch and affection, and relief of pain. In the first stage of life, the infant's behaviors to get needs met are appropriate and life sustaining; in the last stage of life, these strivings appear uncomfortably noisy, out of control, and undignified. Nevertheless, there is a relentless drive in later life to recapture this ineffable experience of trust that has no words and yet carries the basic promise of life.

More than fifteen years after I last saw Joseph, I became curious about what had happened to him (he was now seventy-seven). I was able to get a message to him through the alcohol treatment center where I remembered he had worked as a volunteer. Several days later I heard a familiar voice over the phone; it was Joseph. I reminded him about our work together, which he recalled fondly, and I asked him how his life had been since that time. What I discovered both relieved and amazed me: *Joseph had gotten better.* In the years since our last meeting, he became a respected tribal elder as well as a spiritual counselor for individuals with substance abuse, leading his family, his people, and many suffering addicts through ceremonies that bestowed faith and hope. Joseph returned to the reservation and reclaimed his family's ancestral land. He built a home and planted on his land, and he acquired a small herd of buffalo. He commented on his life's work by saying that the language of the spirit consists not of words but of symbols, ritual, and ceremony. True healing, he discovered, can be found only by going to this deeper level. The vision of Standing Buffalo that had sustained him for so many years was now a living reality on his own land. His life had come full circle, and age had brought him the peace and respect accorded to elders in Lakota culture.

As we finished our phone conversation, I heard Joseph calling to his wife, asking her to remind him of the name of the spirit now assigned to his own grandson, a marine on his way to Iraq. The spirit of Joseph's own grandparent carried him through Korea; now he would support and inspire his grandson in Iraq, as he would his fifty-six other grandchildren scattered around the United States. And what spirit still carried Joseph? "One of the ways we address God," he told me, "can be translated from the Lakota language as meaning *something in sacred motion*. And we know that everything is not stagnant—everything is in motion, and everything is connected." Joseph Red Hair was also Joseph the elder, the healer, and the holy man. In his old age he had discovered a timelessness to the connections among us, a spiritual force beyond the confines of words, of age, and of oldness, accessible to every generation. This was still his guide: "Just be present and open all of the doors around you. Allow the natural spiritual vibrations to come into you and heal you."

Old Pickled Brain

Every old brain has a tale to tell. Sometimes the ravages of age are apparent on simple visual inspection of the organ when it is lifted from its slotted seat in the skull and placed in the pathologist's brine. The serpentine grooves between the aged folds of the brain, once closely pressed together like the fisted fingers of a baby, are now separated by large gaps and channels and resemble the withered meat of a walnut. Remnants of previously robust elastic blood vessels appear as hardened tendrils. Many specimens contain evidence of small strokes and tumors. A slice of brain from any level or lobe, stained and prepped for the microscope, reveals numerous small plaques of toxic amyloid protein surrounded by a debris field of dead neurons.

Mr. Summerhill had such a brain, I imagined, an old brain pickled by years of heavy drinking that at one point crested at a bottle of whiskey daily. I couldn't see the actual brain, mind you, but meeting the seventy-five-year-old man himself made the point all too clearly. His wife had finally had enough of his drinking and threatened divorce one evening, triggering an episode of madness in which he ran around the house ranting and raving and threatening to kill both of them. She called the police, and they hauled him off to a nearby emergency room, where he calmed down, sobered up, and then suffered a seizure after thirty-six hours without imbibing his routine brew. It also turned out that he had been taking massive doses of an antianxiety medication, and now the receptors in his brain had revolted without their daily fix. A neurologist saw him and started an antiseizure medication. Shortly thereafter, the extremely wealthy Mr. Summerhill, now rendered homeless by his wife's restraining order against him, was spirited out of the hospital by his attorney and arrived on the doorsteps of our rehabilitation facility.

I found him ensconced in his one-bedroom suite in the VIP wing of the facility, surrounded by a retinue of personal assistants and attorneys. His secretary, Betty, was gathering and arranging papers for three suited attorneys, while his butler and driver shuttled drinks and snacks into the room. Mr. Summerhill, or Alvin as he requested I call him, was extremely cordial and even deferential when we met. "I hear you're a Harvard man, as am I," he informed me, "and I also have a medical degree from your alma mater." In fact, I noted somewhat suspiciously that most of the staff were referring to him as "Dr. Summerhill." He was dressed in baggy gray sweatpants and a neatly ironed blue tennis jacket, and his gray hairs were remarkably well coiffed for a man who had just spent several days in a hospital. His muscular build surprised me, as it resembled that of a much younger man.

The entourage was impressive, but Summerhill was having a hard time maintaining his polished demeanor. One minute he was sitting calmly, whereas the next he was snarling at his staff and threatening to fire them. Several minutes later he would turn smiling to me and his attorneys and answer questions in a seemingly logical but completely false way, what we refer to in psychiatric lingo as "confabulation." The old pickled brain was trying its best to stay on course, but ironically the absence of alcohol and prescription drugs had unleashed a growing beast. With each passing hour Summerhill grew more hyperactive, grandiose, erratic, and inappropriate.

His attorneys pressed me for a quick solution, knowing that they could never settle a multi-million-dollar divorce case with a certifiably crazy old man. "But what if he *is* crazy?" I questioned them, trying to blend in with their less-than-legal slang. Their responses ignored the growing reality of the moment: "He can't be—just fix him." I decided that the rehabilitation wing was no place for a manic and possibly demented man with a serious drug and alcohol addiction, and so I arranged for him to go to a high-class substance abuse treatment center for the elderly in Palm Beach.

As he was preparing to leave, Summerhill's mind was gyrating out of control. First, he fired—*again*—his entire staff. Second, he asked us to summon his three sons from around the country. "Money is at stake!" he roared. "We'll see who loves me best!" He then asked me if the ambulance could bring a young woman to play with his penis on the way to Palm Beach. "Alvin, I would recommend that you *not* ask that," I implored. "OK, good advice," he said, and then ten minutes later turned to the attractive female EMT, "Will you play with my penis?" She suppressed a smile, hoisted the patient onto a gurney, and answered curtly, "Time to go, Mr. Summerhill." "That's *Doctor* Summerhill!" Alvin replied with a perverse grin.

❊❊❊

Look into the brain of even the most mentally impaired young person, and, barring any recent physical trauma, you'll see a relatively normal-sized brain without anything that betrays its derailed functioning. We still know precious little about what actually is occurring in the brain to disrupt thinking, mood, and behavior, and much of what we do know is extrapolated after the fact. It was the survival of numerous head-injured soldiers during World War I that accelerated this knowledge, because we knew where they'd been hit and how they acted afterward. Damage to the frontal lobe produces changes in judgment, motivation, and language function. Damage to the occipital lobe located in the back of the brain brings changes in visual perception. But such localization of brain function tells only part of the story, because most of our abilities are spread throughout the brain, and higher-order ones, such as consciousness and compassion, lie somewhere beyond our understanding.

Seventeenth-century French philosopher René Descartes subscribed to the belief that our true God-given spirit resided in a small organ in the middle of the brain called the pineal gland and somehow exerted its ghostly vapors therein. "Ridiculous!" we scoff at such beliefs, but with what do we replace them? We speak not of "vapors" today but of "chemical imbalances" that we cannot see but can only infer from stained slices of rat brain or deduce from the fact that boosting levels of chemicals such as serotonin or dopamine in the brain has profound effects on mood, behavior, and perception. The terms and techniques have become more sophisticated since the days of Descartes, but we are still wrestling with the same question of how a human mind emerges from a gray blob of brain matter. Contemporary philosopher John Searle has tried to answer this question with a simple formula. Mind and brain, he asserts, are not two separate things but one in the same, such that "all mental phenomena, whether conscious or unconscious, visual or auditory, pains, tickles, itches, thoughts, in deed, all of our mental life, are caused by processes going on in the brain." This is true for young and old brains alike.

※※※

Summerhill's brain had a rough course in Palm Beach. Though he was sober, having been off both booze and antianxiety meds for several weeks, his memory lapses and hyperactivity were worse. Increasing doses of antiseizure medication, mood stabilizers, antipsychotics, and, eventually, lithium were brought in to dowse the cerebral fire, but with limited success. When I visited him at the request of his attorneys, he was insistent on leaving and returning to his apartment. "But your wife has a restraining order against you," I reminded him. "To hell with her!" he bellowed at me. "I'll sneak in and get what I need!" These moments of willfulness worried me the most. His poor judgment and paranoia could get him into serious trouble, and he had vast financial funds to fuel such trouble. I suggested to his attorney that a legal guardianship was needed before Summerhill, left to his own devices, brought catastrophe on himself and others.

After my visit to Palm Beach, I didn't imagine seeing Summerhill again, but his absence turned out to be a brief respite from a coming storm. After being discharged from the Palm Beach facility, he bounced between one son's house in northern Florida and several five-star Miami hotels, all the time in the company of his secretary, butler, cook, and team of attorneys. I now understood how the eccentric and obsessive-compulsive billionaire Howard Hughes used to get by without ending up in a psychiatric institution. With enough money and staff, a person can call the shots, no matter how insane she or he may be. And so it went, for a while at least, with Summerhill.

One night I received a call from a hospital in Orlando where he had been admitted after having some form of either stroke or seizure. "Was he drinking?" I asked the ER physician. "No, his blood alcohol level was nil." It was becoming clear that I was the only one who really knew Summerhill's history, and even in his fog Summerhill recognized this and made it known to every doctor he saw. "Was he taking his medications?" The ER doc called up the lab results—the blood levels were all in range, except one. Summerhill had apparently taken a few doses of ibuprofen, which pushed his lithium level into a toxic range, resulting in slurred speech and muscle jerks. Lithium is perhaps the best mood-stabilizing medication available, but it is also the most toxic, having a narrow therapeutic window below which it is useless and above which it is deadly. Summerhill was the last person a doctor wanted on lithium, because his impulsivity, poor judgment, and generally uncooperative demeanor interfered with safe monitoring.

I could see where Summerhill was heading. He was sober, but years of alcohol and prescription drugs that had kept the lid on an underlying bipolar disorder were no longer in effect, resulting in mania and psychosis. He also seemed to have a mild dementia from the severe alcohol abuse, manifested in his wildly disjointed stories about his past and recent history. And finally, a survey of Summerhill's life history that I gleaned from his three sons pointed to an extremely obsessive-compulsive and narcissistic man whose very personality dysfunction had led to his financial success as a ruthless and detail-obsessed investor. At the same time, his nasty and capricious demeanor took a toll on everyone around him. I feared that without aggressive intervention he would either end up killing himself or someone else, or his slowed, clumsy, and erratic intellect would continue sputtering out until total dementia set in. I did not imagine that his old pickled brain was capable of much else.

I thus reached a point with Summerhill that I had experienced many times before with other older patients, when a doctor must make a decision in the face of supposed fate and futility. Give up and let nature take its course, or leap in and actually do what needs to be done. In practice, this is not the difference between doing nothing and doing everything, as debates on health care seem to imply. It's not the difference between pulling the plug and trying to jump-start a comatose brain. Rather, it's the difference between settling for the achievement of some physical comfort and striving to enable life *and* positive growth, comfort *and* meaning. It's about not giving up.

I conferred with Mr. Summerhill's attorneys, and we brought him back to the rehabilitation facility. They obtained a tempo-

rary guardianship, and I committed myself to going in front of
a judge to support that petition. Despite the long odds, we decided to try to save Summerhill. For myself, I could honestly
say that his wealth was not the issue. After all, I could charge
him only the same Medicare rates I charged everyone else, and
what I earned in a month of treatment was less than what his
attorneys earned in one hour of billable time. For me, this was
about pushing the envelope of psychiatric care and testing my
own abilities to care for someone; it was about seeing if I could
actually pull the brain from the brine.

From the start, however, things did not go well. Summerhill
was demanding, impulsive, and just plain rude. Every other day
he tried to fire staff members. He insisted on smoking cigars in
prohibited areas. He called in his attorneys for endless meetings
during which he would take copious, disorganized notes. As the
guardianship hearing approached, we met with his three sons
to discuss a long-term plan. Summerhill was paranoid about
their intentions. "What do you want of my estate?" he yelled.
"Who loves me most?" he demanded to know. Each son entreated him to be sensible and tried to reassure him of their intentions, but Summerhill was too far gone to understand.
Amazingly, these were nice boys who had somehow survived
growing up with a tyrannical, alcoholic, and manic father.

As the guardianship hearing approach, I tried my best to regulate Summerhill's medications, but they were only poor brakes
on a speeding freight train. Every other day I was being called
for one emergency or another. The final straw came late one
Thursday afternoon when Summerhill and his sponsor from Alcoholic's Anonymous attempted to drive off campus against our

explicit instructions. I was called out to the guardhouse, where Summerhill sat jumping about in the front seat of the car, wide-eyed and enraged over the guard's refusal to open the gate. "Drive though it! Knock it down!" he screamed at his AA sponsor, who sat in the driver's seat, trembling and confused at the scene. I went toe-to-toe with Summerhill. "You've got to stop this, Alvin. It's not safe for you to leave." I reminded him of the scene he had caused at a restaurant another day when he had run out without paying and then had tried to hitchhike barefoot back to his former penthouse. "It's all lies! I will sue you, sue this place, and all of you will go to jail!" Summerhill could be amazingly sharp and intimidating when he was in a fury.

It was time for the nuclear option. I wrote up a form to involuntarily send him to the county hospital for treatment and then called the Miami Police to enforce the order. After an hour of wrangling with an astonishingly patient and empathic police sergeant, Summerhill gave up and walked into the ambulance. That night he hit rock bottom. When his attorney went to check up on him in the crisis unit at the emergency room, he discovered that Summerhill had stripped himself nude and was ranting, weeping, and frenetically pacing around the quiet room in the smeared puddles of his own urine and excrement. Summerhill's madness was in full bloom. Hearing this, I thought of old King Lear's madness over the loss of his kingdom: "You see me here, you gods, a poor old man, / As full of grief as age; wretched in both."

The doctor at the county psychiatric ward was not a finesser with meds. He dropped the Daisy Cutter on Summerhill's brain using a combination of high doses of the antipsychotics Thorazine and Haldol. Within a day Summerhill was calmed, fogged, slightly rigid, and drooling. I gently suggested to his attorney-turned-guardian that we get him to a nearby geriatric psychiatry ward where I could have a colleague pursue a kinder, gentler regimen. Summerhill was three-quarters gone by now, and I wasn't certain who or what would eventually emerge.

✳✳✳

Sometimes the brain in late life hits a tipping point where it can no longer sustain previous levels of intellect and function. At that point the effects of both medical problems and medications on the brain become exaggerated, and a normally innocuous infection of the bladder or even a toothache can cause a rip-roaring delirium. In such a state, coherent speech gives way to babbling; motor agility surrenders to aimless, uncoordinated picking and pinching; and the air fills with hallucinated images of long-lost loved ones, infestations of bug and rodents, or Lilliputian people tumbling about the room. A manic state and a psychotic state in an older brain are similar in the disorganization they produce, often likened to a mental bonfire where the roaring flames toss back and forth like the outstretched arms of a group of frenzied dancers. A doctor's instinct in the case of both delirium and mania—which can exist simultaneously—is to throw everything on the fire to put it out. But the process of smothering the fire can nearly kill what's left of the human within.

The key is to learn when to advance and when to back off, to select the medications and proper doses that help and avoid those that hurt, and to sense when it's time to act and when patience must reign. Doing so is an art as much as a science, but one best infused with an attitude of care and commitment.

Writer Jay Neugeboren, whose brother Robert suffers from chronic schizophrenia, describes the spirit of this enterprise so well. Based on his own observations over the years, Neugeboren describes the ideal approach of a mental health clinician as being a commitment to a long-term relationship, saying in effect, "I believe in your ability to recover, and I am going to stay with you until you do."

✳✳✳

In many cases with older mentally ill individuals, there is tremendous variability from day to day and from medication to medication, often too much to know with certainty which path is best. Summerhill was a particular challenge because he lit up across the entire diagnostic spectrum, from dementia to substance abuse to personality disorder to severe bipolar disorder, and he had failed most treatments. But after following Summerhill for so many months, I could recite his entire history by rote. I had produced the definitive treatise on his life and mental condition for the judge. Intellectually, I knew he was far gone, but emotionally I was still drawn to the case. Despite the long odds, I wanted badly to succeed.

At the geriatric psychiatry ward I engaged the assistance of my mentor and colleague Dr. Stone to retool the treatment plan. We stopped the medicines that were making Summerhill nonfunctional. Instead, we used a long-acting injectable medication that would guarantee both compliance and a reliable blood level of the medication. Once injected into Summerhill's gluteal muscle, the small blob of antipsychotic degraded slowly over the course of two weeks, when another injection was needed. We added on top two oral medications that would augment the first by rebalancing the chemical neurotransmitters in the brain that we believe lie at the heart of bipolar mania and psychosis without overwhelming the circuits. After several weeks Summerhill was calm, alert, and conversant. He was still somewhat stiff and slowed, but the trade-off was necessary for the time being. We had clearly pulled him back from the brink. Over the course of several months Summerhill became more mentally engaged. He behaved appropriately at the guardianship hearing, and the judge decided to hold off on a permanent guardianship. Summerhill was free, but under close supervision. He agreed to work closely with me to get better.

Over the next year something remarkable happened. Summerhill's mania, psychosis, and cognitive impairment began to evaporate. He attended AA and maintained his sobriety. He returned to my office weekly for counseling and medications, and his impulsive, inappropriate, and self-centered demeanor subsided. After his divorce was settled, he found a girlfriend and began to cultivate near-normal relationships with his sons and their families. The boozing, pill-popping, deranged Summerhill who had swaggered through the social and financial corridors of Miami for several decades was no more. One of my most impaired patients became my most compliant. Though the financial meltdown that hit the country nearly wiped out most of Summerhill's cash reserves, he endured and adapted. Out of the fog his intellect reemerged, and a man who a year prior I would not have trusted to safely walk across the street was driving, managing his finances, and seeking out new ventures.

To this day I still marvel at Summerhill. Once the bipolar disorder and substance abuse problems that had plagued his entire adult life, twisting his personality into a Frankenstein monster of a man, were resolutely treated, a normal older man emerged. With time, the old pickled brain, chemically rebalanced and freed from years of mind-numbing toxins, turned out not to be so pickled. The resilience of the Summerhill brain reminded me of a stunning discovery in 2008 when pathologists studied the donated brain of a Dutch woman, Henrikje Van Andel-Schipper. Her brain was not merely old; it was the oldest brain in existence at the time of her death that year at the age of 115. Such a brain would normally be riddled with pathological findings. But not so with this old brain; in fact, it appeared remarkably normal, with almost no evidence of any age-related changes beyond what would be found at about age 75. These findings corresponded to Van Andel-Schipper's normal performance on standardized neuropsychological tests conducted at the age of 112.

Not every old brain, of course, will be in such terrific shape. And not every older individual with the mental illness of a Mr. Summerhill can be salvaged. But there are always the promise and the possibility if we at least try to find them. My patient and friend Mr. Summerhill knows this well, and he instructed me during our last appointment to write his case down for posterity. I promised him I would try.

Lousy

It's only a guess, but something must have happened in the tank. It was December 1944, and a bitter winter had settled over the Allied forces in the Ardennes Forest in Belgium. A furious and unexpected German offensive punched a large bulge in the American and British lines, inflicting heavy casualties on both infantrymen and Sherman tankers. It may have been the threat of or even the actual explosive graze of a menacing *Panzerfaust* charge against his tank or perhaps the terrifying whine of incoming rockets from the *Nebelwerfer*s. Whatever it was, James was never the same. I was able to gather a few facts from a yellowed note in his chart at the veterans hospital dating back to 1945: He was first hospitalized in England for severe nervousness and vomiting, diagnosed with shell shock, and while in the hospital refused to take off his helmet.

Curious thing about the helmet but explainable: What was once called shell shock or war neurosis but is now called post-traumatic stress disorder involves several characteristic symptoms, including hypervigilance, intrusive flashbacks, and avoidance of any stimuli that trigger a state of panic. For James, as with every combat-related PTSD sufferer, part of his mind still lived on the battlefield. The helmet was a necessary accoutrement.

Somewhere along the line, however, James managed a truce with these memories, discarded the helmet, and moved on with his life, marrying twice, fathering two sons, and finding gainful employment as a meat-cutter. When I first met him, he was a seventy-eight-year-old widower who had retired from a large supermarket chain and was living alone in a small suburban house. Although he still had a designated service connection to the VA hospital for "neurosis" that guaranteed free treatment, he had avoided any contact with psychiatry for decades. He came to me reluctantly, then, suspicious about my intentions and insisting that he was only doing his internist a favor. His complaint was clear and about as nonpsychiatric as it could get: "I've got lice."

A year before our meeting John had appeared at the VA emergency room with a bloody nose and complaining of headache and dizziness. These symptoms were attributed to high blood pressure, and he was sent home on a higher dose of a diuretic—*and* with a prescription for a bottle of Kwell shampoo. "Shampoo?" I questioned him. "Oh, yes, I needed it *again* for the lice," he told me. He claimed to have recurrent forms of lice, or "lousiness" as he called it, using a more antiquated diagnostic term no doubt learned in the service. According to James, these lice were infesting his scalp and eyebrows and had spread to his entire body, causing terrible itching and red, oozing sores. He believed that he had acquired them from a less than sanitary barbershop and from "bedbugs" at his cabin in the woods. As proof, he pulled up his sleeves and revealed scattered red scabs in groups of three. Over the past year he had tried multiple prescriptions and over-the-counter medications, but without relief. His medical chart indicated that he had come to both the VA emergency room and the urgent care clinic on many occasions with the same complaints: itching, headache, tingling, skin lesions, and concerns about seeing lice flying around his house.

This was my first clue that something was amiss: *Lice don't fly.* And even if they did, they certainly wouldn't be biting someone's skin in groups of three. Pediculosis, as it is called, is a human parasitic infection caused by the tiny blood-sucking ectoparasite *Pediculus humanas*—or louse—a small, *wingless* crawling creature with six legs, two antennae, and retractable needlelike jaws. *Pediculosis capitis* is the most common form of infection, in which lice live and lay their eggs, or nits, in the scalp, causing intense itching and excoriation. There are also variants that infect the body and the pubic region. At the time I saw James the main form of treatment for lice was a onetime application of Kwell shampoo and ointment, which contain a neurotoxic insecticide called lindane.

It was clear to me that pediculosis was not the true diagnosis here, but rather that James had a somewhat rare and incredibly treatment-resistant form of psychosis known as a delusion of parasitosis or Ekbom's syndrome. These individuals are well known to dermatologists, presenting with diffuse complaints of itching and crawling sensations in their skin and with visible self-induced skin excoriations—sometimes secondarily infected—that they attribute to some form of parasite. Most of the time the sufferers of this particularly virulent delusion go from doctor to doctor seeking help, sometimes bringing in small vials of "bugs" that actually contain small pieces of dried, scratched-off skin. They are often smart enough to know, as James figured out quite quickly, that the antipsychotic agents given to them are *not* dermatologic medications used to treat lice.

My concern with James was not so much with his skin or even with his delusion. I was more concerned with the myriad neurological symptoms he was reporting, including headaches, tingling, dizziness, and memory lapses, and the fact that he was practically bathing himself in a neurotoxic shampoo and ointment on a frequent basis. In addition, every day he was spraying his hat, clothes, bedsheets, and furniture with an antilice spray that contained another neurotoxic insecticide. Although nowadays Kwell is considered a second-line treatment for lice due to concerns about its potential neurotoxic and carcinogenic properties, it was for James the treatment of choice given to him by half a dozen doctors over the course of a year—most of who did not realize what their colleagues were also doing.

The treatment could have been worse, I thought, knowing that previous approaches to the eradication of lice included the application of DDT powder to body and clothing or the use of other poisons containing derivatives of cyanide or mercury. The aggressive use of these obviously toxic agents had to be weighed against the fact that the common body louse was historically considered a vector for lots of nasty diseases, including typhus and trench fever. Even though I knew that James did not have to worry about such diseases, I also realized that part of him was still sitting petrified in a Sherman tank during the Battle of the Bulge, believing that the "flying lice" attacking him, like the Nazi scourge, had to be eradicated at all costs. In his mind it was "kill or be killed," and if that meant greasing up his hat, or helmet, with lindane or some other toxin, well that's what a good soldier had to do.

After a few sessions I built up enough trust with James to convince him to try an antipsychotic agent, casting it as a way to improve his sleep and lessen all of the stress he felt over his "infestation." I implored him to stop using all of the insecticidal ointments, shampoos, and sprays, telling him in stark terms that they could kill him. I referred him to a colleague in neurology, who thought it was likely that the neurotoxic insecticides were causing his various symptoms. I posted notes in James's chart, contacted all of his doctors, and even called the pharmacy he frequented, begging everyone to restrict his access to antilice products.

My notes over the ensuing year were telling. James claimed to be taking the antipsychotic agent, but he also claimed that the lice infestations were coming and going. "I still see the eggs," he told me one month. He appeared noticeably thinner over time and was slower in speech and movement. He lost his driver's license after passing out at the wheel. I called his son Bill, with whom he had intermittent contact, and expressed my concerns. Bill sighed over the phone and concurred: "I know," he said, "but my Dad will do what he wants do in order to stay safe in his own mind."

Surprisingly, James always kept his appointments with me, punctual to a fault. Other patients missed appointments now and then, but James never did, and so when he didn't show up one morning, I grew concerned. I called the VA van driver, who reported that James hadn't come out of his house at the usual time. James's phone rang repeatedly when I called, but without response. By early afternoon without word from James, I called the police. About an hour later I got a phone call back from an officer informing me that they had found James lying in bed, deceased.

What killed James? I still wonder. Was it his heart? After all, he did have both diabetes and heart disease. Or was it the antilice poisons that were probably still coursing through his skin and nervous system and permeating the fibers of the hat he kept matted to his head on most days. I don't know. But when I think of James's death, I recall the famous words of General Anthony McAuliffe during the Battle of the Bulge when he refused an order to surrender to the surrounding German troops: "Nuts!" he responded. McAuliffe and his men survived the siege of Bastogne because of the determination of Sherman tankers like James, who broke the back of the German lines several weeks later. But a part of that battle lived on, lingering in the helmet, hat, hair, and mind of James, and might have even killed him fifty years later. This, for many old soldiers, is the legacy of war.

The Strange but True
Case of Dawson da Vinci

I have learned in my practice as a geriatric psychiatrist to observe two key maxims. The first has become a cliché in every textbook: Start low, go slow, but *go*. Whether a doctor is dispensing advice, engaging in talk therapy, or prescribing medications, an older patient requires an approach that is moderate, measured, and persistent. The second is based on an old adage in medicine that instructs the doctor to treat the whole person who has the disease rather than just the disease itself. It's a reminder to the practitioner that every disease has a context that is much wider than simply a list of symptoms. Old age is certainly one key consideration, as are factors such as diet, gender, family history, daily habits, and attitude toward illness. Thus, depression in an eighty-five-year-old meat-eating, Irish Catholic, male, World War II combat veteran who loves to exercise will be different from depression in a ninety-year-old, widowed, grapefruit-juice-drinking, retired, female Asian seamstress who is a devout churchgoer. Depression—like every other form of mental illness in late life— is a coat of many colors whose expression and treatment course are fundamentally influenced by all of these unique aspects of the individual.

There is a particular category of mental illness, however, that appears to defy both maxims. In this category, the very being of an afflicted individual as expressed in daily behaviors, attitudes, and emotions is itself considered the disease. We call these mental illnesses *personality disorders*, and they are marked by a pervasive and dysfunctional weirdness, hostility, volatility, self-centeredness, or avoidance of others, to name a few symptoms. These disorders in both young and old are the scarlet letters of psychiatry, and they run roughshod over any concerted and organized attempts at treatment. And when seen through the prism of age, their appearances may be so disruptive and noxious that they appear to strip away all the individual differences that we weigh in the case. I have tried diligently, however, to understand and engage with these older patients, to liberate the person from the label.

※※※

"You are not a Michelangelo!"

I wasn't sure at first whether this declaration from my patient was a true insult or merely an observation. Mr. Dawson, the seventy-eight-year-old patient in question, continued: "You are probably in the 325 range. But I am, on the other hand, a Leonardo da Vinci." Seeing the quizzical look on my face, Mr.

Dawson dug through a jumble of papers on the tray in front of him and retrieved one particular page entitled "The Biometric Cosmos." An inverted pyramid was outlined on the page, balanced on top of another pyramid, and each was divided into subsections with various names and labels and a numbering system ranging from 0 to 800. I could see that the highest category on the top pyramid was labeled "Masters of the Cosmic Gamma," and it included da Vinci's name. I could also see that the category assigned to me by Mr. Dawson was several echelons below his, lying between "Persons incapable of true reason" and "Golddiggers." That didn't sound too complimentary. It could have been worse, though, as the levels below me went from "Unskilled workers in ultraviolet light" to "Imbeciles and Morons" and eventually to "Dust."

Mr. Dawson had been given a number of different labels from the nurses: strange, bizarre, skittish, obnoxious. He was not well liked. I realized, quite quickly, that this was nothing new for Mr. Dawson; over the years he had earned many similar labels in his encounters with staff at the VA hospital, all culminating in the more parsimonious diagnosis of a schizotypal personality disorder. The schizotypal individual is, by definition, an odd character who is uncomfortable with social relationships. Older schizotypal individuals can pose enormous challenges when they arrive, often unwillingly, in clinical settings and refuse to cooperate with standards of care. These strange patients cannot be avoided, however, and are a lot more bearable when understood.

I was asked to evaluate Mr. Dawson after his nurses reported that he was refusing his medications and threatening to sign out against medical advice. He had arrived at the hospital several days earlier with a gangrenous loop of intestine, and following emergency surgery had developed a rapid heart rate, which necessitated a transfer to the cardiac care unit. When I first went to see him, Mr. Dawson was lying in bed with the covers pulled up to his chin and a surgical cap bound tightly to his head, having obtained it after days of arguing with the nurses. I was greeted with a suspicious stare, and the reception only got chillier when I introduced myself as a psychiatrist.

"I consider myself above psychiatry," he stated, "and I don't need the heart doctor either—I have the heart of a twenty-year-old." Despite his antagonism toward psychiatry, Mr. Dawson was interested in talking about his work once I got him on the subject. "I am an evaluator," he described, "and a scientist." He claimed to be a master of evaluating the "cosmic energy" that flows as part of the life force. Handing me the diagram of the biometric pyramids along with another strange scale of "emotional tone," Mr. Dawson outlined, in grandiose terms, his ability to use both energy waves and handwriting samples to evaluate people using a special "box" at his house. And because he was at the level of da Vinci, he claimed that he could evaluate someone just by looking at the person. I asked him why he was in such a hurry to leave the hospital.

"First of all, I am not psychotic. But you have to understand the unseen forces here. The nurses send vibrations towards me but do not accept mine in return. This imbalance has caused my heart to misfire."

Mr. Dawson spoke to me coherently, even eloquently. There was no evidence of cognitive impairment or depression. He was irritable when describing his idiosyncratic demands (e.g., that he had to wear a surgical cap to keep his brain warm), but he was not particularly angry or anxious at other times. He didn't want to be around staff because he was suspicious of their motives and believed that they were causing his problems. At first listen, his thoughts sounded delusional, but as he continued to relate his work to me in such a detailed and rational way, even producing charts prepared by an actual "Biometric Society," I realized that they were—despite their grandiosity and implausibility—more odd than psychotic. After all, some individuals believe wholeheartedly in clairvoyance or astrology—why not the "biometric cosmos"?

For most of his life, Mr. Dawson had had neither the desire nor the fortitude to spend much time around others. He did not report disliking people, but he clearly did not feel comfortable in their presence. He was somewhat autistic in his approach, not being able to actually read the emotional tone of others (despite his self-described status as an "evaluator") or separate out his own emotional feelings from the reality of the environment. Though he was intelligent, he clearly demonstrated a warped interpretation of the behaviors of people around him. Over time Mr. Dawson had increasingly withdrawn from social contacts, grown suspicious of others, and developed a number of unusual interests and mannerisms. Eminent personality researcher Theodore Millon describes this process as a crucible for schizotypal personalities, in which "the more individuals turn inward, the more they lose contact with the styles of behavior and thought of those around them."

The further consequences of this isolation and the lack of social feedback from others are that schizotypal individuals "gradually begin the process of acting, thinking, and perceiving in peculiar, unreal, and somewhat 'crazy' ways." These patterns are not in essence psychotic, even though the general schizotypal personality may spin off brief psychotic episodes and share elements with a psychotic disorder such as schizophrenia. It is widely believed that schizotypal traits do not change much with aging but become more entrenched—as was the case with Mr. Dawson. By the time I saw him, he had a lifetime of odd beliefs and behaviors woven into his character.

Like many individuals with late-life personality disorders, Mr. Dawson also demonstrated other enduring and pervasive dysfunctional traits: schizotypal, obsessive-compulsive, paranoid, narcissistic, and passive-aggressive. Put together, these traits composed a man who was isolative, yet pompous, seeking to flee from the hospital, yet seemingly drawn to the presence of others who indulged his desire to talk about his work in excruciating detail. In the end, however, he was resisting and even sabotaging efforts to help him, and he was leaving everyone around him feeling angry, confused, and even frightened. Up until being hospitalized, he had retained his independence and hadn't needed to interact much with others. But now his age and medical condition demanded help and forced him into situations that he could handle only in his typically odd and hostile manner.

It is tempting to dismiss the late-life course of many older individuals labeled with chronic mental illnesses. In this scheme we focus instead on the "personality disorder" or the "schizophrenic" or the "demented" as if they were no more than a stereotyped disease. We open our treatment manual, and it spells out a clear formula of psychiatric evaluation, medication, and, oftentimes, institutionalization for each category. Being old and being mentally ill are a double whammy, bringing derision and discrimination from two different directions. Even the doctors who tend to these individuals face discrimination in terms of reduced and highly limited insurance payments and thus salaries.

In the end, Mr. Dawson signed out of the hospital against medical advice but agreed to follow up with both a cardiologist and my clinic within the week. I wasn't optimistic, because individuals with schizotypal traits can be notoriously difficult to engage in any form of psychotherapy. I wasn't surprised either when he refused to consider any medication, but I was disappointed. There is reasonable evidence suggesting that the use of low-dose antipsychotic medications in his case could improve symptoms of paranoia, thought disorder, hostility, anxiety, and even obsessive-compulsiveness that are commonly associated with the schizotypal personality.

I figured that even without medications Mr. Dawson would do best when he wasn't forced to be around people and would return to his eccentric pursuits. I remained concerned, however, about whether he was able to take care of himself, especially because he refused his cardiac medications, asserting that he knew better than the doctor. This is where clinicians often clash with schizotypal patients, becoming annoyed at their poor adherence to treatment and assuming that they are psychotic and incapable of making clear decisions. That assumption, however, is not necessarily true. In most cases decisionmaking is relatively intact though intransigent, and we have no choice but to accept their ways and their decisions, no matter how strange they may seem.

Mr. Dawson was a no-show for the appointment, and so I asked the clinic's social worker, Dan, to make a home visit. I warned Dan ahead of time that Mr. Dawson—the self-styled da Vinci—might appear and act quite strange and fill him with lots of bizarre theories of the cosmos: "Dawson da Vinci claims to actually practice with some form of a biometric box," I added, "but that is likely not true."

"Not so," Dan informed me later that day. As it turned out, there *was* an actual biometric box in Mr. Dawson's apartment, an eight foot by twelve inch square polished wooden box with a metallic meter in its center and a silken cord attached to a small woolen cap at one end. Mr. Dawson even gave a demonstration, having Dan place his hands on the box while Dawson wore the cap and appeared to enter a brief trance. He rated my colleague with a gamma score of 420, meaning that he was a "true individualist"—almost approaching the level of Galileo!

"Strange," Dan commented, giving me a wry smile, "but true!"

Part III
Memory

*My history falls away, like sacks of grain from a
careless farmer's wagon. I begin to forget everything.*

—JOSEPH SKIBELL, *A BLESSING ON THE MOON*

If I Forget Thee

Emily was a pleasant, bespectacled woman of eighty-two years who guided herself into my office at the controls of her electric scooter. I was impressed by her careful maneuvering around the desk and assumed, prematurely, that she must be cognitively intact. But when I asked her to tell me about herself, she was befuddled. "You're not the eye doctor?" she queried, "because I need my glasses fixed." I explained my role again and asked her about her memory. "It's okay," she said, "no better, no worse than average." She recounted her history, but with many gaps. When I asked her how many times she had been married, she stated, "Two or three times." I persisted: "Was it two or three marriages?" She didn't remember and conflated two names into one. Her first husband, she thought, had died in the war. Or was that the second? I tried to imagine the missing men here, no longer even memories to Emily, just faint traces of "someone."

Alzheimer's disease was slowly engulfing her brain, and soon even Emily's notion of marriage would disappear. Place and time were fading as known entities to her, aside from the clear road directly in front of her scooter. With time, even her own name would slip away, taking with it her identity and those of all the beloved people in her life. Perhaps the only consolation would be her inability to even know whom to mourn.

Seeing Emily, I wondered about the consequences of losing such defining memories and was reminded of the oft-quoted passage from Psalm 137 in which the Hebrew exiles in Babylon cry, "If I forget thee, O Jerusalem, let my right hand forget her cunning. If I do not remember thee, let my tongue cleave to the roof of my mouth." For these ancient exiles, the imagined price of forgetting a beloved memory was a paralysis of sorts involving the loss of both physical and verbal functioning. In some respects, Emily and other aged individuals suffering from progressive dementia face a similar exile from the memories that once defined their identities. And with time they lose their very ability to act and communicate in meaningful ways.

This evolving exile is depicted quite poignantly in sequential self-portraits by artist William Utermohlen created throughout the first five years of his suffering from Alzheimer's disease. Compared to a detailed sketch of his healthy appearance from earlier years, a painting done two years after his initial diagnosis reveals distortions in both the shape and symmetry of his face along with a bewildered and anxious expression as the disease creeps in. Three years into the illness the colors of the drawn face become starker, the artist looks utterly confused, and the entire head is disembodied and trapped in a rough frame. In year four the facial expression has disappeared into a maelstrom of white and green, and the head is floating in a box with an enlarged, misshapen ear. The last portrait in year five is primitive and bereft of color, consisting of a round swirl of pencil lines with two dotted nostrils in the center. The identity is absent in this last drawing, but a trace of sensory awareness remains. By his midseventies Utermohlen had stopped painting.

The end result of dementia seems wholly tragic, a premature death in which all of the lines, shapes, colors, and memories that built a lifetime of love, purpose, and meaning have been wiped away. And this tragedy is compounded when the losses are exploited. Consider how often we discuss the conditions or behaviors of cognitively impaired individuals in their presence, assuming that they cannot understand what we are saying. I once witnessed a particularly cruel example of this exploitation when serving as a consultant at a Boston-area nursing home. A couple who had been married for more than seventy years shared a room at the facility, each suffering from severe dementia and largely unaware of the presence of the other in the adjacent bed. One morning the husband passed away, and within hours of his body being removed from the room, a new roommate was put in his bed. The widow lay silently nearby, unable, it seemed, to take notice or utter any complaints. The administrators of the facility believed that the newly widowed woman was unaware of her loss and acted without regard for her dignity. They were embarrassed and contrite when confronted, yet did nothing to prevent a future occurrence of such disrespect to a resident.

In the face of a memory disorder, then, how can we respond to the relentless loss of persona inflicted on its sufferers? We can acknowledge the tragedy and grieve the lost identities and memories, but is there anything more substantive to be done beyond maintaining the individual's physical presence? To the administrators of the nursing home, the severely demented widow was little more than a body in a bed, waiting her turn to be replaced. Most of us would not knowingly act in such an uncaring manner, but instead we may have a more passive—but equally uncaring—approach. We simply ignore, avoid, or neglect our most debilitated elderly. The problem with nursing home placement is not the placement itself or the fact of having to live in a nursing home; the problem is the abandonment and the loneliness visited on those so placed. But these are human-made problems, not products of age. The exile, then, may be twofold: exile from memory and exile from memorable, caring people. But is there anything we can do to help these exiles come home?

My patients have taught me two lessons. First, it is easy to miss sparks of the person hidden under the burden of disease. I once interviewed a ninety-five-year-old man with moderate dementia who was unable to provide much history due to his memory loss. The day was late when we finished our meeting, and I decided to take him in his wheelchair across our campus to his room. On the way we happened across a friend of his, whom he greeted warmly in Russian and with whom he carried on an animated conversation. At one point they switched to Polish, then to Yiddish, and they ended up in song together as they linked arms. For my patient, the words and cadence of a first language were like the inspiring taste of the madeleine cookie for Marcel Proust, reawakening memories and skills that flowed as naturally as in the past.

Second, we can step in to discover and even help rejuvenate the person behind the lost memories. I saw a powerful example of this role with my patient Hannah. I had first met her about ten years previously when she was a caregiver for her husband, Edwin, who suffered from Alzheimer's disease. Several years later Edwin passed away, and Hannah began to demonstrate signs of memory loss herself. I remained her doctor and referred her to a special social club for individuals with early-stage dementia. Hannah's identity revolved around several pillars: her beauty, her exile from Poland and then Cuba, and her dedication to social service. Even as she lost more and more of her independence, she struggled fiercely to maintain her dignified manner and dress. She also retained a fair amount of insight into her illness and often reported feeling depressed by her memory loss.

Then a generous neighbor stepped into Hannah's life and offered to make a scrapbook for her. With Hannah's help, the neighbor prepared a laminated book that included a narrative of Hannah's life, photos of her as a young woman in Poland and Cuba, and copies of certificates and newspaper clippings that recounted her involvement in the community. All that Hannah had difficulty remembering could be found in this amazing book, and she carried it with her everywhere as a reminder of who she was. It was astounding to see the restorative transformation in Hannah as she proudly showed the book to others. The scrapbook became, in essence, a portable identity.

I would like to think that even in the last days of dementia there are still traces of memory that allow patients to keep someone in their hearts. At the long-term care facility where I work, the music therapist, Joseph, was once working with a ninety-three-year-old severely demented woman who would sit in a wheelchair all day and make a repetitive clicking sound with her tongue. No words, utterances, or grunts—just clicks. After several hours of this noise she would become an extreme annoyance to staff and residents alike. Such repetitive vocalizations are always difficult to treat, and as her doctor I was having almost no success. More often than not, the medications that quell such vocalizations work only when they have sedated the person—a wholly unacceptable prospect.

Fortunately, Joseph had a better plan than I did, and so one day he brought the woman into a music therapy session. As Joseph played on the keyboard, each participant kept the beat in her or his own way. One older man shook a tambourine, while another tapped a small drum. Meanwhile, the old woman just clicked away. Several of the other residents were getting distracted and annoyed and began to yell at her to shut up. As Joseph listened to the woman's clicking, however, he began to sense a rhythm; "Click, click-click, click click-click." Something familiar struck him, and he began to play out the rhythm on the keyboard. As he played, a song began to fall into place, and the woman took notice. With more notes, the song became clearer, and her clicking suddenly ceased, her eyes opened wide, she took a deep breath, and she began to sing, "Let–me–call–you–sweetheart!" These were the first words anyone had ever heard her speak.

Joseph kept playing, and the woman kept singing—"I'm–in–love–with–you"—while the rest of the group sat in stunned silence, their pieces of percussion momentarily silenced.

Joseph later learned that "Let Me Call You Sweetheart" had been the song played so many years ago at the woman's wedding with her beloved husband. Ever since, it had always been "their" song. Even in the depths of dementia, one fond memory persisted, without words or tune and likely without images, only a rhythm indelibly imprinted on a clicking tongue.

I am also reminded of an elderly female patient with severe dementia who was visited daily by her husband. He doted on her, providing attention and affection even though she no longer remembered who he was. When he died unexpectedly, I witnessed this same woman wandering the floor in tears for many weeks, no doubt feeling deeply grieved over a missing presence. She had no memories of what she missed, but a part of her brain instinctively felt emotions that her caregivers were able to recognize and soothe. When her daughter and grandchildren visited with her several weeks later, there were no more tears, just embraces and laughter. They were able to help restore a small part of what had gone missing.

Fortunately, dementia is not a universal affliction of age. Being "senile" does not mean being demented; it simply means being "old"—although too often the terms are used interchangeably, and we end up equating aging with memory loss. We must realize, instead, that for many older individuals aging brings a vast repository of memories that carry with them the identity and history of the person and of the larger society. An eyewitness to history can impart memories in ways that books cannot.

The process of recalling the past, known as reminiscence, is a particularly powerful and vital activity in late life. In his autobiography, author and Holocaust survivor Aharon Appelfeld describes how "ever since my childhood, I have felt that memory is a living and effervescent reservoir that animates my being." In reminiscing about his own life, Appelfeld explains, "memory and imagination sometimes dwell together. In those long-buried years it was as if they competed. Memory was tangible, as if solid. Imagination had wings. Memory pulled toward the known, and imagination sailed toward the unknown."

This interplay between memory and imagination may explain the dreamlike quality to memories of the past, which Appelfield experiences as both "elusive and selective" in their conjuring. It is not always clear how and why we come to review certain events over others, but there is always the potential for memories to change how we look at life and for us, in turn, to overlay the memories with new meaning. Such a possibility exists in the very way our brains process memory. Sensations and events are registered and reviewed in a small snail-shaped part of the brain called the hippocampus. The most powerful memories, whether pleasant or traumatic, are imbued with strong sensations and deep emotions by a separate almond-shaped bundle of neurons called the amygdala. For example, most of my older patients can recall exactly where they were and what they were doing when they learned of the Japanese attack on Pearl Harbor on December 7, 1941, because it was such an emotional event. This type of indelible recollection is called a "flashbulb memory" because it sits almost like an exact photograph in our minds and can be easily recalled and reviewed with voluminous detail and emotion. For those and other less dramatic events, the brain prioritizes, encodes, and then spreads them like interlinking spider webs throughout its various regions.

This makes them easier to recall because there are multiple avenues of contact. The entire process, known as consolidation, forms our permanent long-term memory stores.

It is tempting to view these long-term memories as permanently shaped channels in the brain, but research indicates that they are more malleable than previously thought. When recalled, memories become like softened gels that are then reremembered or reconsolidated back to their hardened forms by neurons that reactivate the connections between them. In the softened states, however, we can change these memories by actually altering the attachment of emotions and meaning. This process may account for how individuals with post-traumatic stress disorder can be healed slowly through rote and repetitive verbalization of their traumatic memories, leaving some of the painful emotions and sensations stripped away with each retelling.

Gerontologist Robert Butler was the first person to propose a greater therapeutic role for reminiscence, or "life review," as he called it. He felt strongly that the life review process was both natural and healthy and could help aging individuals revisit and come to terms with unresolved conflicts. Tapping into remote memories and long-held beliefs as well as current thoughts and self-observations could provide an individual with a sense of continuity and strength, especially during times of rapid change or loss. Under ideal conditions, he proposed, life review held the promise of bringing increased "candor, serenity, and wisdom."

The process of life review is facilitated by several factors in late life. First, individuals may have more time for self-reflection, and second, they often face losses and stresses that trigger the need to tap into past life skills in order to cope. A number of psychologists have also proposed that the way in which we organize and think about ideas changes in adulthood in ways that support the goals of life review. Theories of cognitive development are traditionally based on the work of Swiss psychologist Jean Piaget, who proposed that a certain endpoint is reached in young adulthood with the achievement of "formal operations," a stage characterized by abstract thinking and the ability to formulate and test hypotheses. However, the concept of *post*-formal thinking posits that aging adults can develop beyond this stage, acquiring the ability to examine and balance the needs of competing relationships, systems, or perspectives. For example, postformal thinking allows an individual to balance logic and emotion in decisionmaking and to see how he or she participates in creating perspective. Life review thrives on this expanded view of reality as it allows for greater patience, acceptance, and pragmatism in complex situations, whether present or past. This is exactly the skill that Butler and others refer to as "wisdom."

Unfortunately, reminiscence can also reactivate traumatic memories and even trigger depression in other aged individuals. A life review may only highlight mistakes or losses or be rendered useless by denial, distorted or grandiose recollections, or memory loss. Other individuals may be able to acknowledge past transgressions but feel hopeless about the possibility for forgiveness. Still other individuals are too paralyzed by daily life to even engage in the process. In *The Life Cycle Completed*, Joan and Erik Erikson describe how "in one's eighties and nineties one may no longer have the luxury of such retrospective despair. Loss of capacities and disintegration may demand almost all of one's attention." As a result, life review may fail to keep despair at bay in the last, or ninth, stage of life.

Life review, then, carries with it the potential for both rejuvenation and reconsolidation of past memories, as well as the risk of retraumatization. For many of my patients, however, any talk of past events may initially seem pointless. There is often despair that no one will listen, or if they do listen, they will not care. I have learned, then, that life review is not meant to be a solo trek and that any risks can be mitigated when memories are shared, guided, or even shaped within a relationship with another caring and interested individual or even with an audience. Writing an autobiography can also serve this purpose.

This fact struck me after reading *Living in the Shadow of the Freud Family*, written and edited by Sophie Freud, a distinguished professor emerita of social work at Simmons College and granddaughter of Sigmund Freud. Sophie Freud's book is both a family history and an autobiography set within the annotated diary of her mother, Esti Drucker Freud, who was married to Sigmund and Martha Freud's second child and oldest son, Martin. It is a unique form of life review that presents memories, elaborates on them through several voices, and then tries to gain some understanding of their meaning after many decades of reflection.

Esti Drucker Freud's memoirs begin by recounting her childhood in Vienna in the early years of the twentieth century, followed by her courtship with Martin Freud while he was a soldier in the Austrian Army during World War I. After the war they married and had two children, Walter and Sophie, but their ill-fated union quickly began to break apart as economic and social pressures increased in the days leading up to World War II. Sophie Freud adds her own fascinating commentary and queries: "Do happy memories disappear in a generalized glow, while unhappy memories remain much sharper?" This question persists throughout the entire book as the story seesaws among the memories, many soaked in sadness and tragedy, of several generations of parents and children.

After the German invasion of Austria, Sigmund Freud, with international help, received seventeen exit visas enabling his immediate family to emigrate. Sigmund, his wife, his sister-in-law, daughter Anna, son Martin, and grandson Walter fled to England, separating from Esti and Sophie, who traveled to Paris. Shortly thereafter the Germans invaded France and entered Paris, and Esti and Sophie escaped in the nick of time on bicycles, heading first to Nice, then to Casablanca, and finally to the United States. Unfortunately, not everyone in the family made it to safety. Esti's mother, Ida, was caught in southwest France and sent to die at Auschwitz. Several of Sigmund Freud's own sisters were interned in Theresienstadt and then sent to the gas chambers of Treblinka.

Included in this rich life review are Sophie's recollections of her grandfather. As a young child she would visit his famous home at 9 Berggasse in Vienna most Sundays and have a brief audience with him, although these contacts were both limited and formal. "I knew him only superficially and learned about his life mostly through his numerous biographies," laments Sophie. She last saw her grandfather briefly in June 1938 in Paris, where the family had stopped en route to London. Despite physical separation, Sophie was able to have a particularly fond correspondence with him in the ensuing fourteen months before his death in September 1939.

In one letter dated October 26, 1938, Sigmund wrote to Sophie, "I don't answer you as often as you write to me, but be sure to write if you have special experiences or if you need something. I take pleasure with each of your letters." This was a kind appeal to his fourteen-year-old granddaughter, and its impact reverberates over a great expanse of time. At age eighty or so Sophie penned an updated response, which she includes in her book:

> *My Dearest and Much Loved Grandfather,*
>
>   *Even now, in my very old age as I read your loving letters . . . I am deeply moved. Perhaps you really did care about me. . . . I was a child who craved your affection. . . . I remember you as old and sick, with your fingers in your mouth, always in pain, a grandfather of few words. Our visits in your sacred office were short—*

Sophie continues by recalling a walk in the garden with her grandfather while collecting nuts: "I knew that this was a rare and precious moment, a moment of pure joy, to be ground forever into my memory." She thanks Sigmund for the loving letters that he wrote her in the year before his death, seeing them as proof that he cared about her.

I decided after reading this extraordinary book to seek out Sophie Freud herself. I had actually met her many years back at a psychiatric conference in Boston, and so I was familiar with the great work she had done in the field of social work over the course of her long career. I made contact, and Sophie invited me to visit her at her home in the woods outside Boston. When I arrived, she greeted me warmly and expressed satisfaction that I had correctly navigated the serpentine roads to her driveway. This exciting visit felt a little bit like a pilgrimage to a holy seer by virtue of her eighty-five years and her role as a living, genetic extension of Sigmund Freud. After all, the very foundation of my life's work as a psychiatrist, including the vast majority of everything I had ever read on human nature, was shaped by her grandfather. Even so, Sophie was not Sigmund, and I had come to hear her own thoughts about aging and memory, and not those of her grandfather.

We sat together in her study, surrounded, floor to ceiling, by books, papers, paintings, and small artistic knickknacks from her life, including a miniature bronze bust of her famous grandfather. The floor of the adjacent living room was covered with a richly detailed red, orange, and blue Oriental rug reminiscent of her grandfather's iconic couch. A nearby computer was in active use, and I was impressed by her facility with both e-mailing and downloading files. Outside of the large sliding glass doors lining the wall of the room was a serene view of her wooded lot, which led down to a small pond. Over the course of several hours she spoke to me about her life, past and current, and insisted that I stay for lunch, tea, and homemade strudel.

We began by speaking about her book. Sophie acknowledged that the eight-year process of writing it had served an important function during the time she was cutting back her full-time work schedule. As she writes in the introduction: "The book project helped me with this difficult transition. It gave meaning to my suddenly senseless life; it has become my closest friend in these somewhat solitary years." The project took so long, in fact, that Sophie worried "that my age would defeat me before I could finish its conception—thus it was a race between a piece of work and my aging brain, in which my drive to work, trained through many years, did win after all." That her "aging" brain could accomplish such a task counters the view that "old people are no longer educable" espoused by Grandfather Freud. "There is often *more* change" in late life, Sophie emphasized to me, "and an enormous need for change and adaptation more than in earlier years."

Even though Sophie is extremely active for her age, she sees herself as much less involved in the world compared to previous years. On the one hand, she continues to teach and take courses at the Brandeis Lifelong Learning Institute, write poetry and short stories, exercise, spend time with her children, and keep up with correspondence. On the other hand, she no longer works full-time, travels around the world, or raises young children as in years past. She still has the sentiment of an activist but not the physical energy: "I've become more of a bystander," she told me, "but I am still sensitive to the suffering that goes on around me." These sentiments were well captured in a recently published poem by Sophie, entitled "The Old Woman and Time":

Was it only yesterday
Or ten years ago
I stood on one foot
straight as a tree

in my yoga class.
Arms over head
saluting the sun
This is so easy. I thought
I could stand here all day.
Today time's typhoon
threatens to blow me down
as I stumble along
on both feet.

During our visit, I asked Sophie about the particularly poignant and intriguing "Apologia" (best described as a defense of her philosophy) in the beginning of her book. There she speaks quite candidly with the reader about aging for her mother and for herself: "Mother, dying of cancer, complained that there was no one in her life who would make her a cup of tea. 'You should have made friends when you were younger,' I said. 'I had no time for friendships,' she responded. 'You always wanted to be left in peace . . . ,' I reproached her, 'and now you are paying the price of such a choice.'"

Her words in this Apologia are honest and harsh and signal to the reader that the book will not hesitate to examine feelings all around. Sophie continues: "In the 20 years since my first book, in this time of my own aging, I have come closer to Mother. She no longer appears so alien to me; I too want to be left in peace. . . . I live alone and now and then I feel alone. Others see me as an eccentric old lady. Many cadavers of cutoff relationships litter my life. I also might not have anyone preparing me a cup of tea when I am sick. Well, there are always electric teapots one can rely on."

I felt a degree of sadness when I read this opening passage, as it seemed to describe Sophie as someone who deliberately sought isolation. And yet the book is incredibly inviting and intimate with the reader. In person, Sophie herself could not have been more personable and hospitable. When I commented on this contrast between her words and her demeanor, Sophie responded with a smile: "I am more independent than most people I know. I need less company because I have my books, and the courses I teach. I did not have to give up my identity as a teacher . . . [and] I do not experience loneliness." Her comments reminded me of the sentiments expressed many years prior by Henry David Thoreau, in whose beloved Walden Pond Sophie swims every summer. When asked by a friend whether he was lonely out in the woods in his cabin, Thoreau responded, "This whole earth which we inhabit is but a point in space. How far apart, think you, dwell the two most distant inhabitants of yonder star? . . . Why should I feel lonely? Is not our planet in the milky way?"

In retrospect, I see how my own ageist assumptions crept in here, imaging that being alone in late life implied loneliness and sadness. But this is certainly not the case for Sophie—and for many other aged individuals. She treasures her solitude and her independence, but they do not preclude interpersonal connections. At eighty-five she is more connected to others than most of her peers. She has a timeless vitality. And my visit allowed me to understand firsthand the spirit that lies behind her written life review. As Sophie herself writes, "This book is the magic bastion Mother has bequeathed me to combat futility in my old age."

I learned an additional lesson about the powerful role of memory in late life from the title of her book—*Living in the*

Shadow of the Freud Family. Among the dozen definitions of the word "shadow" that appear in the dictionary, two in particular have seemingly opposite meanings: A shadow may represent an obstruction of light by some object, and it can serve as a place of hiding and safety. I see memories playing these same roles for so many of my patients. When painful or even traumatic, they blot out much of an individual's identity, obscuring happier memories and engendering a sense of failure, danger, and despair. Sophie herself made this observation within her mother's memoirs.

But so many other memories are like Appelfeld's imagination: They take wing and prove both soothing and elevating as they conjure people and places from the past that bring affirmation of the greatest connections and joys in life. This, of course, is the ultimate goal of reminiscence—not to restore what has been lost but to experience the gratitude that can come only with the realization that we never truly lose the gifts from the most important figures in our lives. Sophie reaches a similar conclusion in her letter to her grandfather, written when she herself had attained his final age:

> *Dearest grandfather,*
>
>   *Being your grandchild has stamped my life. You were a kind and protective presence in my young life, even if emotionally distant . . . but altogether your mighty shadow has enriched my whole life, rather than curtailed it. It was my good fortune, my enormous privilege, to be born your grandchild and I thank you for all you have done for me.*
> *Your Sopherl*

Savant, of Sorts

Everyone has a photographic memory.
Some don't have film.

—STEVEN WRIGHT

What does the number thirty-seven look like? Most of us visualize two black-and-white numerals side by side, but Daniel Tammet sees an image that he likens to lumpy porridge. After suffering from severe seizures at the age of four, Daniel developed a condition known as *synesthesia*, in which two or more senses are experienced together. He "sees" numbers as shapes full of light, color, and texture, allowing him to perform incredible calculations by seeing the numerical landscape in his mind. On one occasion he memorized the number pi to 22,514 digits and recited them without mistake over the course of five hours. In another jaw-dropping challenge, he studied Icelandic—one of the most difficult languages for a nonnative speaker to learn—for only one week before going on national television in Iceland and stunning the audience by being interviewed live in its native language. Daniel has what is known as the "savant syndrome," which is characterized by the innate possession of spectacular mental skills, such as being able to memorize massive lists of numbers or statistics, quickly learn new languages, or instantly perform complex mathematical calculations.

Imagine how different the world would be if we could simply look at or listen to something just one time and then remember it in its entirety. Like Daniel Tammet, the great composer Wolfgang Amadeus Mozart was believed to have this ability. One legendary story holds that at the age of fourteen Mozart went to the Sistine Chapel to hear a performance of the *Miserere*, a mass whose musical notes had been kept secret for nearly a century. Afterward, he retired to his room and transcribed the entire piece from memory! This skill has been called photographic, or eidetic, memory. Despite the numerous people who have demonstrated this ability, some memory researchers have argued that photographic memory does not really exist, that individuals who appear to have eidetic memory are actually using memory techniques. One example is retired Japanese engineer Akira Haraguchi, who on October 4, 2006, recited by memory 100,000 digits of the number pi over the course of sixteen hours. To accomplish this task, Haraguchi had spent years practicing a memory technique in which he translated a string of numbers into symbols, which he then used to create memorable stories and poems. During his sixteen-hour feat, he was actually reciting the memorized stories in his head and translating them back into numbers. But even the use of this technique begs the question, How did he remember all of those stories? That ability in itself reveals a spectacular memory.

Unlike Mozart and Tammet, neither my friend Gerald nor I have innate savant abilities. Like Haraguchi, however, we resolved to learn several memory techniques to use in our own daily lives and to teach to some of the individuals at an assisted living facility who were struggling with mild memory lapses. Gerald himself is just over eighty, and as a gerontologist he has been interested for several decades in positive approaches to aging. He had watched me grow my memory assessment clinic for some time but felt strongly that something was missing. "My friend," he instructed me one day, "it's time for action." This meant doing more than simply diagnosing memory problems; we had to engage patients in activities to pump up their mental muscles. Increasingly, research has supported the obvious point that regular cognitive exercises can improve a variety of mental skills, ranging from memory processing speed and retention to visual tracking and fine motor speed. But for countless aging adults facing a general slowdown in cognitive speed and efficiency, the benefits of mental exercise (as opposed to physical exercise) are only now being recognized.

Our first "Memory Fit" class included about a dozen individuals ranging from Susan, a seventy-two-year-old former social worker who wanted to avoid the memory problems she had witnessed in her mother, to Victor, a ninety-three-year-old snowbird and retired stockbroker from Brooklyn who spent his winters in Miami. Gerald and I cotaught the four-week course, with each session featuring a different category of items to remember: names, lists of things and topics, and numbers. We first taught and then practiced with the group a technique to remember names using stimulating mental associations. "I now remember Susan's name perfectly," exclaimed Victor after a little practice, "because her eyes remind me of my niece Susan." We then taught the Roman room technique, in which a list of items is memorized through the creation of a visual image of walking through a familiar house and seeing each item placed in a different room. This mnemonic technique was originally developed and perfected by ancient Roman orators who had long speeches to remember but lacked the teleprompters, PowerPoint slides, or even paper note cards utilized by modern-day speakers. Finally, we had a session to teach ways to break down long strings of numbers and letters into more manageable chunks and then add creative associations. "I finally remember that my license plate number is JR2845," explained Susan, "because I think of belonging to the *Jr.* Women's League from the ages of *28* to *45.*"

As we were reviewing the course material during the final session, a debate over technique erupted. Victor was illustrating to the class how he always knew where he kept the TV remote: It was tethered to a bright yellow carved wooden duck that he pulled out of a bag and ceremonially placed in the middle of the table. "That's not a memory technique; that's a prop!" called out Sam, a ninety-year-old retired travel writer and World War II veteran sitting at the table. "A prop, so what?" Victor fired back. Sam sat up ramrod straight in his chair and began to deliver a short speech. "Dr. Agronin, and Gerald, with all due respect, you have tried your best to teach us these special memory techniques. But in the end, it's too much work. I have a better solution that works for me." Sam reached into his shirt pocket and pulled out a small spiral bound notepad, then continued speaking. "Whatever I need to remember, I just write it down here," he explained, holding out the notepad for all to see. A furious debate ensued, with Victor claiming that the memory techniques were necessary and Sam insisting that keeping a written list was more practical. Within minutes the debate became Talmudic. "But how many notepads do you need?" queried Victor, "and what if you lose the notepad?" Sam thrust his hand in the air, pointing toward Victor's shirt, "You will only lose the notepad if you forget to wear a shirt!" Victor was not convinced—"but my shirt has no pocket!" At this point Gerald and I jumped in. "Whatever works for each of you is best," we counseled. "Victor's duck, Sam's notepad—they both work!"

The course taught me several key lessons about memory. I started out as a teacher but finished as a student, realizing that any chronically busy multitasking individual, whether doctor, patient, student, or senior citizen, can suffer from memory lapses. Research clearly shows greater declines in memory with age, including a higher frequency of "tip-of-the-tongue" experiences, but it is equally true that training and practice can significantly improve performance, rendering some of the age-related differences meaningless. In addition, the aging brain has two advantages over younger brains: a lot more experience (and hence, a larger knowledge base) and a greater ability to see both sides of the coin, better known as wisdom. If you are comparing yourself to someone like Haraguchi, however, do not despair. Simply having an awesome memory doesn't guarantee success, as you still need "street smarts" to know how to apply it. After all, even Mr. Haraguchi once forgot his wife's birthday!

My own memory test occurred a year after completing the course. I had just finished giving a lecture on memory to a group of residents at the assisted living facility when a familiar face stood up in the back of the room. "I have a question," my former student called out. "What's my name?" I had just lectured on the importance of practicing several memory techniques, and now my snowbird friend from Brooklyn was testing me. I hesitated for an uncomfortably long pause. A few associations triggered by my former student's heavy accent tumbled from the recesses of my memory: Brooklyn, sea, fish. Fish! . . . Tuna? Cod? Haddock? And then it came to me. I smiled and reached out my arm. "Welcome back to Miami, Mr. *Herring!*" I called out. Victor smiled knowingly, a small notepad bulging in the front pocket of his shirt.

Strength in Numbers

We have all seen a flock of birds or a swarm of bees, but what about a *parliament* of owls? Or a *shrewdness* of apes? According to James Lipton's wonderful compendium, most animal groups have terms that, to a greater or lesser extent, capture the meaning of the collective. These terms might be based on certain characteristics of the animals, like a *leap* of leopards or a *knot* of toads, or on some early linguist's onomatopoetic attempt to capture the sound of the animal, as in a *gaggle* of geese. And what about human groups? Lipton suggests, to our amusement, that we might encounter a *flush* of plumbers, a *wince* of dentists, or a *void* of urologists. He even dares to propose that a group of psychoanalysts might be termed a *complex*! Whatever we call it, when people who have a common mission or plight get together, they form a stronger unit that is able to achieve on a level far above that of the individual.

So it is with memory disorders. I encountered such a group recently when I was invited to give a talk on the brain to twelve ladies who all faced a similar dilemma: Suffering from early-stage Alzheimer's disease, they were too impaired for many senior activities in the community, yet not impaired enough to benefit from the average day care program for individuals with more severe forms of dementia. To meet their needs, I worked with my staff to create a special social club designed to emphasize skills that are resistant to early-stage memory loss, such as imagination, sensory enjoyment, and camaraderie. Led by a group leader with training in memory disorders, the ladies in the club had lectures on humor and history; they read poetry, listened to music, and sang; they read a selected book and had discussions on the content; and they sat together in a leisurely luncheon to talk and laugh about whatever topics came their way.

My invitation to lecture to them on the brain was accompanied by a list of ten questions that the participants had devised the week before and inscribed on a chalkboard. My arrival was greeted enthusiastically by the group, not because they knew me as a particularly wise lecturer, but because I was their doctor, having evaluated each and every one prior to enrollment in the program. I knew their deficits well, having reluctantly conferred their very diagnoses. When they saw me in the clinic, these ladies were typically friendly and gracious but reticent, sobered by the exposure of their cognitive deficit in my presence. Individually, I rarely get many questions from them; they listened intently to my words and often turned to an accompanying husband or adult child for assistance and reassurance.

Meeting with them as a group, however, I encountered something quite different. I saw broad smiles and heard small talk that easily gave way to giggling or burst into full-bodied laughter. They did not merely ask me about the brain; they interrogated me with ten of the most sophisticated questions on brain function imaginable. How do the right and left hemispheres differ? they asked. Do male and female brains think differently? The questions flowed logically from one to another, and as I spoke, group members jumped in to discuss my responses, add in their own commentaries, and pose thoughtful follow-up questions.

Alone, each member of the group faced a growing sense of disconnection from personal memories and other aspects of her identity. Together, however, they shared not just a common ailment, but also common aspirations to feel a part of something larger than themselves, to feel loved and cared for, to care for someone else, and to laugh in the face of adversity. They interacted in ways that defied their individual limitations, with their strengths united. As I talked about the wonders of the brain, I concluded each of my responses to the ten questions with the same theme: Although short-term verbal memory may wane in the face of numerous age-related diseases, our brains have many different ways to capture life experiences, yielding a vast storehouse of persistent memories and cognitive skills. The goal of our social club was to tap into these latent skills, and as I lectured, I witnessed an extraordinary demonstration of these brain powers in tandem with others—a true strength in numbers. And what would I call this group? I recall a sketch from Lipton's book that depicts a dozen beautifully choreographed larks flying together—an *exaltation* of larks, a phrase that gives the book its very title. That is what I saw in the group that day—a joy, a dignity, a strength, and a true *exaltation* of friends.

Old Soldiers

D-Day, June 6, 1944. H-Hour + 15 minutes, 6:45 AM. Uncle Red Sector, Utah Beach. Members of the U.S. Army's 359th Infantry Regiment, including a young private named Clarence Green, hit the Normandy beaches in the third wave of attack. Several miles to the east, another young soldier named Jake Custer of the famed "Blue and Grey" 29th Infantry Division was welcomed to the hell of Omaha Beach in the early hours of the attack. Both soldiers, now in their eighties, have vivid recollections of the events of that day. It was their first time in battle, their first witness to death. Clarence recalls the intense seasickness and stench of vomit in the Higgins boat as it neared the shore. Jake remembers charging onto the beach, hearing a deafening explosion to his right, and seeing nothing but the limb of a buddy fall nearby. Several days prior, however, their spirits had been quite different. Only nineteen years old, they were full of bravado and anticipation, having no true idea of what they would face in the coming invasion. War historian Stephen Ambrose describes how young men who had never experienced the carnage of warfare had a sense of invulnerability, so much so that one young soldier, informed that likely nine out of ten soldiers would be casualties of the D-Day invasion, "looked at the man to his left, then at the man to his right, and thought to himself, You poor bastards."

In circumstances of war, such massive denial serves a function: to enable headlong, impulsive acts that, if left to older men, might never happen. This form of denial is facilitated by lack of both information and experience, coupled with poor insight into impending possibilities. And it likely has a neurological basis, sustained by not fully matured frontal lobes that allow for the excessive risk-taking, aggression, and impulsivity that are gold on the battlefield.

In the clinic, however, this denial is not so golden. For years after the war, Clarence struggled with emotional outbursts, nightmares, and panic attacks, refusing to accept the possibility of psychiatric illness. This denial was willful but not calculated and was enabled by the same ignorance and poor insight that had once sustained his warrior mind-set on the eve of D-Day. Although for a doctor such denial can be problematic, leading a patient to refuse treatments for an illness not recognized in the first place, it can itself be corrected.

There are other forms of denial that are not so amenable to correction. These are cases in which the core mechanism is not lack of understanding or anticipation but a state of forced or innate inattention. In other words, the patient cannot help it. Trauma to one side of the brain, for example, can cause an individual to ignore or even deny the existence of the paralyzed side of the body opposite the lesion. In some individuals, the loss of integrity of their basic body image turns out to be a whole-brain conspiracy, linking together visual impairments with impairments in attention, motivation, insight, and prioritization. Neurologist Joseph Babinski originally coined the term "anosognosia" to describe this syndrome, but the word has come to mean a general state of denial of illness.

Given these linkages, patients express their difficulties in many ways: Some individuals merely ignore the paralyzed side, others actively deny its existence, and still others develop a dislike or even hatred for a paralyzed limb. The search for some meaning to the predicament may even lead to overly elaborate or even delusional beliefs about the limb. In "The Man Who Fell Out of Bed," neurologist Oliver Sacks describes just such a case in which he was asked to consult on a man who fell out of bed after pushing his leg out first, convinced that it was someone else's severed leg that had been attached to him in some sort of cruel New Year's Eve joke.

Despite my lack of military experience, I am always tempted to salute Mr. Custer when I visit the Veteran's nursing home and find him sitting in his wheelchair at the front door, wearing a baseball cap with the word "D-Day" scrawled across each side. What I call valor he calls duty, speaking proudly but not arrogantly about his service. Looking back, he neither denies nor is preoccupied with the unpleasant parts of his combat experiences. He is generally satisfied with his life.

Jake Custer's contentment reminds me of a fellow soldier and veterans home resident named Ben, who is in the middle stages of dementia, most likely of the Alzheimer's type. "Do you have any memory problems?" I recently inquired of Ben, to which he resoundingly replied, "Of course not." Like the young Jake Custer predawn June 6, 1944, Ben is in complete denial of his current predicament and impending course. In the moment, he lives for lunch or for a laugh with one of his buddies. Like the current Jake Custer, Ben is generally satisfied with his life, enabled, to be sure, by his dense denial of reality. In this case, Ben's denial is both willful and pathologic, prompted by a laid-back character who never paid much attention to illness and sustained by small lesions riddling his frontal lobes and their grip on reality. He is in denial about his cognitive deficits in the same way that a stroke victim can deny a limb hanging limply. In this case, there is no point to my trying to convince him that he is ill.

Curiously, in dementia different forms of knowledge help guide a person's daily life, some in complete and blissful denial of certain facts, others acutely aware of the surrounding vista. What astounded newsmakers but generated a yawn from most geriatricians perfectly illustrated this fact: Former Supreme Court justice Sandra Day O'Connor's husband, John, suffering from Alzheimer's disease and residing in a long-term care facility, took up with a girlfriend and was acting "like a teenager in love," oblivious to his marriage of fifty-five years. Here we see complete denial of long-term biographical knowledge, yet perfect awareness of erotic emotions not experienced since his early twenties. This phenomenon takes many forms and is an everyday event in most dementia wards.

From the standpoint of the doctor, determining whether denial of illness is willful or pathologic helps guide efforts to convince the cognitively intact person of the necessity of care or, alternatively, to respect the convictions of the denier, yet work around them. After all, war may be hell, but illness does not have to be.

Memories, False and Fixed

Doctor Al, my uncle, calls it "the shrine." He was the second and now I am the third generation of doctors to sit at this old wooden desk, preserved just as it looked back in 1946 when my grandfather first opened his practice. On one side sits an old-fashioned rotary phone, next to the portable blood pressure cuff that my grandfather used to carry with him on house calls. The elegant blotter in the middle of the desk has two raised leather sides, with a yellowed piece of paper taped to the left and containing the typewritten names and phone extensions of the six other doctors who lived and worked in and near the town of Kaukauna, Wisconsin. The drawers still contain patients' note cards, old glass pathology slides, and various medical knick-knacks from a bygone era. Most interesting to me are the two medical texts I keep on top of the desk: *Stedman's Medical*

Dictionary, 10th edition, published in 1928, and James Meakins's *Practice of Medicine*, published in 1936. I look at these timepieces every once in a while, out of curiosity and out of a desire to see how far we've come in medicine today.

The references to psychiatric terms in these two worn leather tomes are particularly interesting. For example, in 1928 the terms "psychopathist" and "alienist" were two common synonyms for "psychiatrist." Attention to political correctness and risk management were not to be found in 1936, as Meakins described chronic alcoholics as "immoral" and "untruthful" and recommended a brew of toxic sedatives, including phenobarbital and sodium bromide, to treat anxiety disorders. Other terms, however, do not yield the same sense of pride and appreciation for how far psychiatry has progressed.

Take the term "psychosis" as an example. According to the 2004 version of the medical dictionary, psychosis is "a severe mental disorder, with or without organic damage, characterized by derangement of personality and loss of contact with reality and causing deterioration of normal social functioning." The 1928 version was not so specific, defining psychosis as "any mental state or condition" and "a disorder of the mind, insanity," having ten different types, ranging from "exhaustion psychosis" to "toxic psychosis." Meakins was similarly broad. I have often noted, however, that these broader, antiquated definitions of psychosis are too often applied to older individuals whose memories seem disjointed or false. When such memories or, indeed, "any mental state or condition" is painted as psychosis, the logical treatment involves relatively potent medications. Here are two illustrative cases.

Bugs

The call from the nurse on duty at the assisted living facility was brief and to the point: "Dr. Agronin, please see Mrs. Nestor and get her started on something—she's *psychotic*." Betty, the head nurse, followed up with another message: "She has bizarre complaints of bugs crawling all over her room and infesting her clothes and skin. Please see her soon."

I was surprised. Mrs. Nestor, or Francine as I called her, was a particularly friendly woman who usually came to appointments accompanied by her daughter Judy and carrying a box of family photos. I knew that her grandson was an aspiring actor and had been elected class valedictorian. One granddaughter loved ice-skating; another had just started college. Francine treated me like a long-lost cousin each time we met, discussing family and friends and recent events with a joy so refreshing in a ninety-year-old woman. But now . . . bugs?

Francine arrived without her characteristic smile or banter and was clearly preoccupied with something. Because the appointment had been scheduled at the last minute, Judy wasn't able to accompany her mother. There was no box of photos. "How *are* you?" I asked.

"Doctor, I am so upset! There are bugs everywhere!" For the next fifteen minutes Francine described to me in detail how small black bugs were coming out of her newspaper and infesting her room. I was struck by how different she appeared in both voice and demeanor as she described the pathways around the room that the bugs were traversing. She pointed out several small spots on her skin that were itching, and she attributed them to the bugs. Her concerns were overly detailed and seemed implausible, suggesting that she actually did have what we call in psychiatric parlance a "delusion of parasitosis"—meaning a false and fixed belief of being infested by insects. In addition, her visual descriptions of the actual bugs were vague and yet made them sound monstrous, suggestive of visual hallucinations. Perhaps the nurses were right—Francine was psychotic!

After my evaluation, I ordered a urinalysis, reviewed her medications, and was poised to order an antipsychotic medication. I didn't trust my own judgment, however. Francine the smiling cousin versus Francine the frightened entomophobe— I just couldn't put the two together. I put down my pen and pad and called her daughter, who was appropriately concerned by her mom's behavior. I acted on a hunch: "Judy, I need to ask you a favor. Before I do anything else, will you inspect your mom's room for me?"

Judy called me back an hour later from her mom's room. She was laughing. "It's infested! There are bugs everywhere!" Francine, I learned, kept her newspapers rolled up on the floor near the window. Ants were entering through the floorboards, crawling out of the newspapers, up along a bead of dried jelly that had spilled on her rocking chair, through her shawl and over her shoulders, and onto her end table, where she had left an open bag of candies. When seen without glasses, Francine's visual impairment made small black ants appear much larger and fuzzier. Several had irritated her skin with small bites, adding to her discomfort. Only someone sitting in her rocking chair could appreciate the extent of the infestation—but the nurses saw Francine only down in the dining hall or the activity room.

I was relieved by the discovery but not surprised. After all, this is Florida, where ants are practically the state animal, and so I should have suspected a true infestation immediately! At the same time, I realized how close I had come to mistaking Francine's recollections for a nonexistent psychotic symptom. But this was a job for an exterminator, not a geriatric psychiatrist.

Switched

I had known Ed Blum for several years because I used to take care of his wife, Shirley. She had suffered from dementia, and Ed had been her main caregiver, informant, and mode of transportation for all clinic appointments. Late into the course of her illness Shirley began to deteriorate rapidly, around the same time that Ed suffered from a bout of pneumonia with an associated delirium. Delirium is an acute form of brain impairment, often superimposed on other illnesses, and involves waxing and waning disorientation, hallucinations, and agitation. Ed was admitted to the hospital for intravenous antibiotics and then moved to the rehabilitation unit at the nursing home. It took about two months for his delirium to fully resolve.

Sadly, Shirley passed away while Ed was recuperating from the pneumonia and delirium. Ed was able to attend the funeral and appeared appropriately grieved at the time. After fully recovering from his medical problems, however, Ed was still quite weak and unable to walk, and his daughter arranged for him to move permanently into the nursing home. Several weeks later a consult request came into my office: "Please see Mr. Blum— he is *psychotic*."

When I saw Ed, he seemed at first like his old self. He was generally well oriented, in good spirits, and cracking jokes: "Doc, did you hear the one about the priest and the rabbi riding in a plane together?" I had not heard that one, and Ed had me laughing a minute later. He told me about his days as a bandleader during the heyday of Miami Beach in the 1960s, playing with Frank Sinatra and other celebrities at the time. I then turned the subject to his present condition, and Ed reassured me that he was adjusting nicely to the nursing home. There was, however, one sticking point. Ed was not convinced that his wife had really died, and he was concerned about where she was.

"But, Ed, didn't you go to the funeral?" I asked.

"Yes, I remember the funeral, but that isn't my wife in the grave. It's my *mother*—they buried her in my wife's plot. A switch was made."

I tried to reconstruct Ed's logic. He knew that Shirley was gone, but he did not remember what had happened to her, and he had no recollection of sitting at her bedside when she died. When pressed, he admitted that his mother had died years before—"I remember *her* funeral!" he told me. Then why, I asked, did he think someone would put his mother's body into a grave marked for his wife? "I don't know," he replied.

When I saw Ed a week later, I asked him again what had happened to his wife. "They tell me that she died," he related, "but I am not certain. I just don't believe it." He was still convinced that his mother had been switched into his wife's plot. When I asked where Shirley was, his thoughts were murky. "I just don't know."

On the face of it, Ed seemed delusional in his belief that his wife had not actually died, and no argument could convince him otherwise. Such a false and fixed belief might seem to be a logical flight from the reality of his wife's death—a delusional form of denial. I also wondered whether Ed had a delusion of misidentification: Was he switching the memory of his mother with that of his wife? Or was Ed merely confused?

I held off giving him an antipsychotic because he was otherwise doing well and was not overly bothered by his belief. In addition, there seemed to be a plausible explanation for this potential delusion. Because of his previous delirium, Ed had only vague memories of his wife's death and burial. He knew only that his wife was gone, and like a good husband of more than fifty years, he was appropriately concerned. It was hard for him to believe what he had been told because he could not truly remember it happening. Ed's "delusion" seemed more like a poorly reconstructed memory from a dream or, in his case, from a delirium.

✳✳✳

Francine's near-miss diagnosis of psychosis raises an important issue that many older individuals face. Lacking a blood test or a brain scan for "delusionality," the diagnosis will ultimately rest on whether the doctor or other health care professional believes in the veracity of the patient's memories or not, which in turn depends on the time and energy devoted to learning the truth. After all, the paranoid person may have a real enemy and the jealous wife may have a true romantic rival. The "Martha Mitchell effect," a term coined by my college professor Brendan Maher, describes a situation in which a mental health clinician mistakenly diagnoses a patient's description of real events as delusional. He named this effect after Martha Beall Mitchell, the wife of Richard Nixon's attorney general, John Mitchell, who was said to be mentally ill when she began reporting to the press in the early 1970s that illegal actions were happening at the White House. The Watergate investigation later proved her correct—but not before she had been vilified by friends and family for her behaviors. Older patients, in particular, are often assumed to be unreliable historians, and many end up—like Francine almost did—being treated for psychotic "symptoms" that don't actually exist.

But with Ed, his belief was patently false. It seems to qualify as a delusion on the basis of the three criteria first outlined by psychiatrist and philosopher Karl Jaspers in 1913: (1) It is a strongly held belief, (2) no argument or logic can convince the person otherwise, and (3) the belief is clearly false to other people. And yet there are many other sorts of beliefs that might meet these criteria, but we would not consider them to be delusional. Jaspers might respond to this concern by pointing out that it is the form of the delusional belief, more than the content, that elicits the diagnosis. Thus, the way in which a truly psychotic individual persists in his or her delusional thought unfazed by counterarguments, contrary evidence, or incredulous witnesses is what leads to the diagnosis. Jaspers also described primary delusions as ultimately un-understandable, meaning that they have no logical underlying context in the person's life. As before, the diagnosis of a true "delusion" in some cases comes down to the point of view of the observer and the depth of the clinical investigation.

Ed's belief might qualify as a "secondary delusion" under Jaspers's scheme, because it is understandable given his mood (he was depressed over his wife's disappearance) and recent history (he attended her funeral). In a classic work on psychopathology, British psychiatrist Andrew Sims uses the term "delusion-like idea" to describe such a belief. As Ed's grief subsides and he comes to grips with his wife's death, he may correctly believe that it is her body, not that of his mother, buried in Shirley's plot. Only time will tell.

Clearly, the 1928 *Stedman's* definition of psychosis encompasses a grab bag of psychiatric disturbances and neglects to account for the extensive writings on the meaning of psychosis by Karl Jaspers and others that were well known at the time. The 2004 *Stedman's* is more specific but still allows for the diagnostic errors and ambiguities presented by the cases of Francine and Ed.

Yet this may explain why I keep the shrine in my possession, with its old instruments, weathered books and pamphlets, and aging medical knowledge inside its drawers or placed on its sturdy wooden surface. Even though my profession has journeyed across many years and successive generations of practitioners, there is still much knowledge to be gained from looking back at where we came from. And much of the wisdom of years past is still relevant today—perhaps waiting to be reawakened with a little time and effort. This shrine—my grandfather's desk—is also a tangible metaphor for the older individuals with whom I work, teaching me that studying the memories from the past is a pathway to enlivening the present and opening a doorway to the future.

Part IV
Wisdom

Days should speak,
and multitude of years should teach wisdom.

—JOB 32:7

The Elders

The summer of 1972 was a momentous one in the history of Miami Beach. In the middle of July the Democratic National Convention convened at the Miami Beach Convention Center and, after a tumultuous week of late-night sessions, selected South Dakota senator George S. McGovern as the party's presidential candidate. The political temper of the time, roiled by conflicts over Vietnam, civil rights, and women's rights, stoked the passions of the delegates and guaranteed that the final result would not come easily. McGovern's determined political team was able to prevail, but only after sufficient balloting chaos among punch-drunk delegates who selected him over twelve other candidates and his running mate, Senator Thomas Eagleton of Missouri, over seventy-six other candidates submitted for voting, including Mao Zedong and Archie Bunker. In a 3 AM televised acceptance speech, McGovern trumpeted the essence of his campaign message: "I am here as your candidate tonight in large part because during four administrations of both parties a terrible war has been charted behind closed doors. I want those doors opened, and I want that war closed."

One month later the Republicans came to the same convention center on Miami Beach to confirm President Richard Nixon as their candidate for a second term. In his acceptance speech Nixon cleverly sought to undermine McGovern's floundering attempts at party unity: "Six weeks ago our opponents at their convention rejected many of the great principles of the Democratic Party. To those millions who have been driven out of their home in the Democratic Party, we say come home. We say come home not to another party, but we say come home to the great principles we Americans believe in together."

Although the pageantry and discipline of the Republican convention far outpaced those of the Democrats that summer, all hell broke loose in the streets. Antiwar protesters flocked to Miami Beach from around the country, where they met a strong police presence and the streets filled with tear gas. Despite a wise and well-intentioned attempt to confine most protests and protesters to a safe zone, Flamingo Park, several blocks from the convention center, the days of the convention saw screaming and aggressive protests against the delegates, mass arrests, and general chaos in the streets. The outcome of the election, however, bore no relationship to the passion of the protests, as Nixon's landslide victory over McGovern was one of the largest in U.S. history.

It has been close to forty years since that hot and troubled summer. Individuals who once struggled as delegates to make the political process more inclusive are now an entrenched part of the establishment. Young protesters of various stripes are now grandparents. Many radicals of that time still push for peace or justice, but their fervor prompts no fears—real or imagined—of violence or sedition. The streets around the Miami Beach Convention Center, a mere fifteen minutes from my office, are quiet. Flamingo Park is serene, with the only strident voices being those of young people running and playing. The poor and gritty streets of South Beach have been transformed into a sheik bastion of Art Deco hotels, boutiques, and clubs. Forty years ago a cross-sectional survey of Miami Beach would have revealed, so the joke goes, that its residents were born as Hispanic males and died as Yiddish-accented Jewish ladies. The senior boom has largely passed, however, with many of them living and dying in nursing homes like the one in which I work.

As a psychiatrist for the old, I am fascinated by the remnants of such a historical time. But the details of what happened as told by its aged eyewitnesses are not the only thing I find most informative. I want to know how they think *now*. How has age changed their perspectives? It is easy to imagine that the passage of time dulls the emotions of the past, softens a person's political bent, and brings greater understanding for past opponents. I saw this reflected in some of the comments on a historical account of the Miami events of 1972 that I found on the Internet: "Looking back there is only one thing I regret in my life," commented one former protester, now nearly sixty, "and that is being conned by the Anti-American Left during my youth."

Or perhaps age brings greater entrenchment of perspective. "I am still a liberal and proud of it," stated another anonymous former protester and Internet commentator, adding that he would still "fight in the streets to end this war." At the same time, a common stereotype is that old age brings less flexibility and greater obtuseness regarding detail. Age brings more experience, that is certain, and likely greater knowledge of things, but do these elements necessarily bring wisdom? And what do we mean by wisdom in the first place?

In the spring of 2008 I brought these questions to a former history professor and Methodist minister who had a particularly keen vantage point during the events of 1972. This eighty-five-year-old retired professor had also been a pilot in the U.S. Army Air Corps during World War II, flying thirty-five missions as a B-24 Liberator bomber pilot and awarded the Distinguished Flying Cross for saving his entire crew in an emergency landing. And what was this man's role during the summer of 1972? He was the man in the middle of it all: George S. McGovern.

I met McGovern in March 2008 when he came to speak at the annual meeting of the American Association for Geriatric Psychiatry (AAGP). As the medical editor for the organization's newsletter, I decided to seek him out for an interview, to which he readily agreed. In my research prior to our meeting, I learned that McGovern had served South Dakota as a congressman from 1957 to 1961 and as a senator from 1963 to 1981. From 1961 to 1963 he worked in the White House as President John F. Kennedy's director of the Food for Peace program.

McGovern's very presence at the AAGP meeting was an exciting event for so many attendees and served as a touchstone of powerful memories for those who had been politically active during the 1972 election. One colleague excitedly told McGovern how as a high school student she had campaigned for him and had had *his* poster on the wall of her room, as opposed to a poster of, say, the Beatles. His loss had been such a blow that she had sworn off any further political involvement. Another colleague recalled working as a medical student at an emergency medical station for protesters during the street riots.

McGovern himself is tall, dapper, and unassuming. He has a quietness and a warmth that radiate compassion and thoughtfulness. He is only a moderately aged version of the middle-aged man who strode upon the Miami stage back in 1972, and he retains the intellectual acuity and formidable orator skills that have characterized his entire career. Today McGovern remains in Mitchell, South Dakota, the town of his upbringing. He lives with one of his daughters ever since the death in 2007 of his beloved wife, Eleanor, after sixty-three years of marriage. Her loss was a body blow that he has only recently begun to recover from, aided by his decision to get back on the road—often traveling alone—to reach out to people and lecture on various topics. He readily admits that the intensity of his grief after Eleanor's death disrupted both his appetite and his normal pattern of sleep. With time, both bodily functions resumed their normal rhythms, but the experience changed his views on aging. He is less concerned now with what he might achieve and more focused on the value of interpersonal experiences. "I'd give everything I own in a heartbeat to have her back for one more year or one day," he said of Eleanor.

McGovern's sentiments echoed some of the dimensions of successful aging articulated by George Vaillant. As Vaillant has discovered through decades of research in Harvard's Study of

Adult Development (which he directs), successful aging is less dependent on the maintenance of perfect memory and cognition than on the "sustained capacity for joy." The study has followed three subgroups of a total of eight hundred individuals since the 1920s and 1930s, providing one-of-a-kind longitudinal physical, psychological, and social histories for these now-octogenarian subjects. Vaillant has found that good relationships are more important than events in terms of bringing happiness and that a good marriage at age fifty predicts positive aging at age eighty.

McGovern has certainly lived these findings. He was known, and still is, for the strength of his interpersonal relationships. Ironically, this may have been his political Achilles' heel in 1972 when up against the ruthless campaign of Nixon and his minions. McGovern recounted the controversy that erupted when it was revealed that his running mate Eagleton had been hospitalized several times for depression and treated with electroconvulsive therapy. McGovern initially rallied to Eagleton's side, even declaring that he was "1000 percent" behind him, despite deafening pressure from fellow Democratic leaders and the national press to dump the vice-presidential running mate. McGovern carefully weighed the pros and cons of keeping Eagleton on the ticket, consulting with multiple insightful individuals, including "America's most famous psychiatrist," Dr. Karl Menninger, whom McGovern managed to reach in a 2 AM phone call. Within a few short weeks Eagleton withdrew as the nominee and was replaced by Sargent Shriver, but not before the entire incident and McGovern's perceived handling of it did considerable political damage and may have contributed to his landslide loss.

I was particularly curious about how McGovern viewed the events of 1972 through the lens of old age. Had it given him a different perspective? "Right now, I think I'd be a better president than I would have thirty-six years ago," he told me. "I've learned more about the importance of working across party lines. . . . As I've gotten a little older, I've found I can work with a broader range of people and be comfortable about it." I wondered aloud about what had led to these changes. McGovern pondered for a moment and then answered, "I think you just come to a practical awareness that you can't just plow straight ahead and the devil take the hindmost. It just doesn't work that way with human beings. You've got to always have some degree of openness and tolerance for opposing points of view. . . . I've even become more eager to read opposing points of view."

McGovern was quick to add that being open and tolerant "doesn't mean you become flabby about where you stand on public issues." Instead, he articulated what has become a defining characteristic of wisdom: "a capacity to see that problems are really complicated, that there are other angles that have to be considered." Such a perspective, which includes self-education about all sides of an issue, leads to different ways of approaching problems: "I don't make snap judgments as quickly as I might have in earlier times," McGovern described. "I do think one characteristic of youth is to be impetuous, to assume that they're wiser than their parents, wiser than older acquaintances. I think I've developed a growing appreciation for the insights of other people."

McGovern's thinking is in line with what both gerontologists and cognitive theorists have discovered about the capacities of the aging brain. In *The Mature Mind*, geriatric psychiatrist

Gene Cohen summarizes the growing body of research demonstrating that aging individuals develop a new ability to think, strategize, and devise solutions in ways that go beyond the abstract, or formal, reasoning that Jean Piaget described as the endpoint of cognitive development. "Postformal reasoning," Cohen writes, "helps integrate the subjective and the objective, feeling and thinking, the heart and the mind, and becomes more facile . . . [in] deal[ing] with conflicting opposites in the second half of life." Psychologist Judith Stevens-Long describes how older thinkers can "integrate logic and the irrational aspect of experience. . . . [They] see not only how truth can be a product of a particular system, but also how the thinker participates in creating the truth." According to these definitions, postformal thinking allows an older individual to look at both sides of the coin simultaneously and then reason without being hampered by the inherent ambiguity or contradiction in the situation. This ability is life sustaining and even *life saving* in the final years.

It's easy to imagine how this sort of thinking comes into play with McGovern and many of his aged peers who continue to pursue meaningful activities even after profound losses. As a younger man McGovern was a war hero who commandeered bombers and a dedicated public servant who served under President Kennedy ("like being around royalty," he told me). As a middle-aged man he stood with the great political giants of our time and counted himself among them. He was one election away from the most powerful position in the world. There were years in which he was one of the most recognized figures on the planet. Yet now he travels alone, carrying his own suitcase through airports and walking about almost anonymously in most settings. Aging has robbed him of his political stature, influence, public recognition, and life companion. His horizon of activity, even with the best of actuarial projections, is measured in a few short years. Many younger individuals project themselves and their youthful sensibility into McGovern's stage and see only futility in front of a closing doorway. And yet for McGovern, this side of the coin doesn't stop him, doesn't haunt him, and doesn't preclude his interest and ability in seeking new adventure.

Indeed, the concept of a postformal mental state embodied so well by George McGovern was envisioned centuries ago by Roman philosopher Marcus Cicero in his famous essay "On Old Age." He wrote that "the reasons why old age is regarded as unhappy are four: one, it withdraws us from active employments; another, it impairs physical vigor; the third, it deprives us of nearly all sensual pleasures; and four, it is the verge of death." Yet Cicero sought to counter these beliefs by asserting that old age should be guided by rational reflection and not by the hedonistic pursuits we value in younger years. "The arms best adapted to old age," he wrote, "are the attainment and practice of the virtues; if cultivated at every period of life these produce wonderful fruits when you reach old age."

Such an approach can help an individual to recognize and cultivate many new strengths and advantages in later life that do not depend on physical vigor or sensuality. In fact, Cicero held that the pursuit of physical pleasures was actually a burden of youth that was lifted in later life. Freed from the youthful intensity of physical passions and girded with knowledge and wisdom, the accrued influence "is the crowning glory of old age."

Like a modern-day Cicero, Cohen writes passionately that the myth of cerebral decline must be countered by the fact that the brain *can* grow new nerve connections and physically resculpt itself in later life. As a result, the aging brain has the potential for more mature and interconnected neural circuitry to regulate thinking, emotions, and creativity. A recent study in support of this hypothesis found that the brains of older individuals are less emotionally reactive when viewing negative images, and another study showed that older individuals have more positive autobiographical recall compared to younger subjects. A large-scale survey published in 2010 found that levels of self-reported well-being and happiness declined from age eighteen to age fifty and then began to improve, nearly peaking at age eighty-five. In essence, aging may enable individuals to increasingly take to heart and brain the notion "Don't worry; be happy." Even though the vicissitudes of aging are always unpredictable, both ancient and modern lines of thought encourage individuals to think and act positively in late life while suggesting that the aging brain is better able to do so.

On this basis, Cohen proposes a series of human-potential phases that "reflect evolving mental maturity, ongoing human development, and psychological growth as we age." In each phase there is a surge of energy that promotes new activities and interests. In McGovern's case, after he lost his Senate seat in 1980, he founded a liberal political action committee, went back to teaching history, and then, in 1984 at the age of sixty-two, attempted another run for the presidency. Such persistent activity represents Cohen's "liberation phase," which occurs from the fifties to the seventies and during which individuals take advantage of newfound personal freedom and creativity to explore new pursuits. At the age of seventy-two McGovern suffered the tragic loss of his daughter Terry to alcoholism. Despite his grief, he wrote a book about her struggle and started a foundation in her name. Then in 1998 he began serving as the U.S. ambassador to the UN Food and Agriculture Organization, and in 2001 he was appointed the UN global ambassador on world hunger, recapitulating his earlier work on world hunger as a young member of the Kennedy administration. These activities occurred during what Cohen describes as the "summing-up phase," which occurs from the sixties to the nineties (and overlaps to some extent Erikson's eighth stage of integrity versus despair and Vaillant's "keeper of the meaning" phase) and during which an individual searches for a larger meaning to life, energized by wisdom and a desire to contribute to the world.

The last phase in Cohen's scheme is the "encore phase," beginning in the late seventies and characterized by personal reflection and reaffirmation and celebration of the major themes in a person's life. McGovern's presence on the lecture circuit, sans entourage, brings him back to his earliest roots as a politician and even a minister, traveling around and lecturing to audiences. He has also returned to his academic roots as a historian with a 2008 book on Abraham Lincoln. In my interview with McGovern, I asked him to sum up his life wisdom: "Be intellectually honest," he advised. "Don't shade the truth. Say what you honestly think. When I ran in '72, I said that I was making one pledge above all others: to seek and speak the truth. And I really tried to do that."

Cohen has described numerous other influential individuals who provide similar evidence for his scheme of aging, such as author Alex Haley, who began in middle age a search for his family history that eventually became the best-selling book *Roots*, and iconic dancer Martha Graham, who from her retirement as a ballet dancer at the age of seventy-five to her death at ninety-six spent her time choreographing new ballets. This incredible potential for artistic creativity in late life is perhaps best exemplified by the many great folk artists producing works (and even starting careers!) in their eighties and nineties. But are these extraordinary elders the outliers? Is such potential accessible for the aging masses?

Cohen suggests the development of what he terms a "social portfolio" to enable everyone to cultivate a sense of meaning, vitality, and dignity in later life. This practical approach is analogous to management of a financial portfolio and begins with an accounting of assets, including an individual's interests, skills, resources, and relationships. The social portfolio intends a slow buildup of assets over time and includes some form of insurance for dealing with potential losses. For example, an individual categorizes personal assets according to individual and group pursuits and then segregates them according to the degree of energy and mobility that they require. A sixty-five-year-old person who loves to ski with friends (a group activity requiring high energy levels and independent mobility) will eventually need to pursue alternative group and individual activities that involve lower levels of energy and mobility. The key is to identify activities (such as hiking, nature walks, bird-watching) that can bring equal degrees of gratification and socialization but are more realistically accomplished. An individual then possesses a list of vital and meaningful pursuits, and the process of developing the portfolio, sharing it with others, and reviewing it over time can motivate and inspire those who might otherwise drift toward stagnation and despair as they age. Keeping these interests in reserve provides a form of psychological insurance, preventing the avid skier from seeing life as less meaningful when she or he can no longer safely manage the same slopes.

Cohen basically defines wisdom as a broadening of perspective that includes the cultivation of creativity and social interaction. Neuroscientist Elkhonon Goldberg looks at wisdom as a product of nerve pathways built up over a lifetime of experiences. These pathways allow decisionmaking to increasingly take the form of "pattern recognition rather than problem solving." In practice, this means that the wise elder can quickly size up a situation and render judgment, almost like the "blink" that Malcolm Gladwell describes in his best-selling book on the subject.

But most longitudinal studies on cognitive ability have shown clear declines in performance starting in the fifties and sixties and encompassing a broad range of skills, including memory processing speed, numerical ability, visual pattern recognition, and word fluency. So here's a paradox: How does the brain lose capacity at the same time it seems to grow in wisdom? This paradox emerged in a conversation I had with eighty-eight-year-old Dr. Bernard Lown, an eminent cardiologist and current professor emeritus in cardiology at the Harvard School of Public Health who invented the cardiac defibrillator. In addition to his fame as a cardiologist, Lown is equally well known for his work as an international peace activist, winning the Nobel Peace Prize in 1985 for his role as cofounder of International Physicians for the Prevention of Nuclear War.

Lown had strong feelings about aging in general. "As you grow older," he told me, "you grapple with issues of age not out of knowledge but out of ignorance because you are ill prepared for it." Lown did acknowledge the fruits of age, which bring "a certain perspective that is not merely intellectual but is an emotional perspective on life—what time is, what sorrow is, and what loss is." And yet as he aged, Lown took notice of declines in the cognitive skills deemed so essential to his role as a doctor. His short-term memory began to atrophy, and the names of drugs or the details of patient histories that had once been at his fingertips became more elusive. "I would engage in circuitous conversation to not let on to somebody that I didn't know it," he said, adding that it became more difficult to keep up with the latest advances in his field. At the same time, however, "I was better in judgment, far better and far keener, and the patients sensed that. They would say to me, 'You're a far better doctor than you were twenty, thirty years ago.'"

As Lown expressed the paradox, he was less sharp on the details and yet somehow better in general as a doctor. But where does this wisdom come from? In part, it derives from the use of cognitive pathways described by Goldberg, where overall decisionmaking has a more automatic quality. It may also represent a shift in cognitive style in which older individuals take in more detail, which slows them down compared to younger people but ultimately results in the retention of more information for later analysis and decisionmaking. In his own words, Lown described acquiring "the ability to commune and perceive an emotional dimension that is pre- or post- or *extra*-verbal. It's not words—it's gestalt. It's an ability to perceive, but more than that, a sensibility to nuance that is so trivial that it is overlooked."

Lown's observations suggest that wisdom may be an emotional skill as much as it is an intellectual one. I thought about this skill when discussing the events of 1972 with Marilyn Gold-aber, who was the director of social work at the Miami Jewish Health Systems when I first began working there in 1999. Marilyn once worked closely with her husband, Irving (now deceased), a sociologist who created and pioneered the use of the "win-win" strategy in which each side in a conflict could emerge with a resolution that met its needs. In fact, it was Irving, working as a consultant to Miami Beach Chief of Police Rocky Pomerance in 1972, who suggested that Flamingo Park be designated as a safe zone for protesters during the summer political conventions. Such a venue gave the protesters a place to camp out and exercise their free speech, while at the same time it relieved the Miami Beach authorities, to some extent, of their fears of the protesters. This certainly wasn't a perfect solution, but one as close to win-win as was possible at such a fractious time.

Today, Marilyn at age eighty-two is as sharp and articulate as she was during the summer of 1972. She now has her new husband, Mac, at her side. Mac is ninety-two years old and appears as fit and trim as the dashing young World War II bomber pilot staring out of the black-and-white wartime photographs in their apartment. He still rises early to exercise and walk five miles, as he has done daily for the last few decades. When I interviewed the couple, Marilyn reported that she was taking aging in stride, but Mac was more resistant. A once compulsively organized journalist and public relations/marketing genius, Mac bemoaned the fact that he could not accomplish even half of what he did when he was younger.

He focused on the decline in his previous abilities and the potential for further calamity. In fact, his description of aging echoed his stories of the Martin B-26 Marauder bombers that he flew on 122 missions in New Guinea during World War II. The plane was a gem once aloft, with great speed, stability, and capacity to drop a devastating payload on its targets. The problem, however, lay in takeoff, when the finicky engines had a high rate of failure at critical moments, earning the plane its nickname as the "widowmaker." "If the engine coughed on takeoff," Mac described, you were a goner because it meant the plane was not achieving sufficient speed and lift to continue climbing. Mac managed a fear of crashing back then, even surviving a bailout into enemy territory in the jungle of New Guinea and a several-week trek alone back to his base, despite being given up for dead by his squadron. But aging, at one point, brought a never-before-experienced lack of reassurance for Mac, who would climb out of bed on some days already burdened by the fear and frustration of potential failure.

During my initial interview with Mac and Marilyn, however, I pushed hard on the issue of wisdom and perspective in late life because I viewed them as role models. "How do you cope with these changes?" I asked Mac. "I don't really adjust," he told me in a tense voice. "I continue to be aggravated. If I make a plan for the day, I stay with the subject, but the problem is now I find myself drifting. I forget the subjects. I lose track of things. And somewhere along the line I find that I'm off the track. I am not meeting my standards." Cognitively, Mac had begun experiencing the slowing of memory processing speed and efficiency that most ninety-year-old brains face. And it seemed to have hit him in a particularly sensitive spot, because mental efficiency had been his trademark since his days in the service.

"Is anything better with age?" I pressed. "Are there any advantages?" Mac resisted the possibility: "I see deterioration on a daily basis" he said. Marilyn, however, chimed in with a different take. "But I see positives," she said, smiling at Mac. "You are much more mellow, much less hard on yourself." Mac had to agree, but he attributed the change to his motivation to please Marilyn or at least not to aggravate her. Marilyn pointed out an increased match between his intellectual and emotional maturity. "Is this different from the relationship you had years ago when you were married to your first wife?" I asked Mac. "I am much more sophisticated now," he confessed. "I know the value of adjusting to the change in my capacities. . . . I realize that if I don't adjust my style and my behavior that I am liable to hurt myself."

Marilyn went even further, describing how Mac had developed rich, loving relationships with his sister and her children that he never had in the past. "He has the capacity he never even knew—*love*," she said. "He is concerned. His sister's as well as my own children and grandchildren adore him. It's a delight. It's a whole life he didn't have. And he has not only adjusted, he's embraced it, and I think he has grown immensely. I see real positive aging." And this positive aging has continued for Mac and Marilyn, so much so that they could barely even relate to some of Mac's original concerns when I sat down with them two years after our original interview to read them excerpts. Even in the short interval between our meetings, they had grown so much as individuals and as a couple. I thought about them later when a ninety-six-year-old patient described how his life had been turned around for the better after working with a therapist on some chronic marital issues. Even at his age and after many years of marital problems and depression, he had found new peace and happiness with his wife.

Herein lies a critical lesson of aging: Even in the context of age-related intellectual decline and other losses, the enhanced capacity to love, create, and renew relationships is a gift of growing old not to be overlooked or trivialized. Surgeon and best-selling author Sherwin Nuland elaborates on this point in *The Art of Aging*, arguing that the factors most critical to successful aging include mutual caring and connectedness, maintenance of physical capability, and creativity. Vaillant's longitudinal data support this suggestion, revealing that the key personal strengths that underlie good relationships in later life include forgiveness, gratitude, and loving-kindness.

In contrast to Mac's embrace of new relationships, previous psychological theories of aging suggested that there was a natural process of disengagement in late life. In truth, many older individuals do have an eclipsed range of personal and social involvements and relationships. This is due in part to the loss of loved ones. Bernard Lown described poignantly how his mother responded to this natural attrition. At the age of ninety-five she asked her son, "Why am I living? I am already dead. The people that defined me are gone, so who am I?" If we are indeed defined by our relationships, Lown points out, then their loss robs us of the energy and memories that keep us going.

But there is a counterpoint to this view. What some see as disengagement may actually represent a pragmatic pruning back of life's activities and relations. This form of wisdom is encapsulated in the work of Laura Carstensen, a psychologist at Stanford, who suggests that aging individuals recognize their limitations and the shrinking horizon ahead and actively place a greater emphasis on seeking more positive and meaningful emotional experiences. The work of Carstensen and others has demonstrated that even in the face of losses such as those experienced by Lown's mother, many older individuals are able to maintain a generally positive emotional state. In my own experiences at the nursing home, it is not always clear whether it is denial, resignation, or acceptance of life's vagaries that enables this mind-set, or perhaps it is something else. This something else may be a form of spiritual wisdom that proves transcendent for many individuals.

During the summer of 1972 at the height of the protests, there was, not surprisingly, a tent in Flamingo Park sporting a handwritten sign that advertised "POT." Numerous young people flocked to the tent, expecting to score some marijuana. They were surprised, even shocked, however, when a young Hasidic rabbi emerged from the tent, proffering not pot but tefillin—the little leather boxes containing Bible verses that observant Jews don during morning prayers. "Put On Tefillin— P.O.T.—that's how I got them to stop by my tent," recalled Rabbi Avrohom Korf, now the Florida regional director of the Chabad Lubavitch organization. In terms of his own spiritual wisdom forty years later, Korf points to the thinking of his own spiritual master, Rabbi Menachem Mendel Schneerson, who held that old age is to be viewed not as a failing but as an ongoing opportunity to accomplish one's purpose in life. For Jews, Christians, Muslims, and people of many other faiths, wisdom, defined as "not merely the result of accumulated information" but as "the ability to focus on the unifying element *behind* all information" represents a call to action. The commandment to "rise up before the aged" (Leviticus 19:32) is not just a call for the young to respect their elders, but for the elders themselves to "rise up before age" and continue to pursue their enhanced ability for spiritual fulfillment.

Twentieth-century theologian Abraham Heschel added an existential component to the notion of spiritual wisdom, suggesting that if late life is "an age of anguish and boredom," then the answer must be to cultivate a sense of significant being as "a thing of the spirit . . . not entertainment but celebration." He added, poetically, that "old men need a vision, not only recreation. Old men need a dream, not only a memory." In this forward-thinking view, aging is a formative time, "rich in possibilities to unlearn the follies of a lifetime, to see through inbred self deceptions, to deepen understanding and compassion, to widen the horizon of honesty, to refine the sense of fairness."

Heschel offered an antidote to the distorted equating of aging with death or dementia that I was taught as a doctor and that permeates our culture. "The effort to restore the dignity of old age will depend upon our ability to revive the equation of old age and wisdom," he wrote. "Wisdom is the substance upon which the inner security of the old will depend forever. But the attainment of wisdom is the work of a lifetime." Wisdom is thus more than an achievement of aging; it is as integral and essential to the aging process as walking is to the toddler, play is to the young child, and the pursuit of love and partnership is to the young adult.

Gerontologist Lars Torstam, influenced in part by Zen Buddhism, elevates the role of spiritual wisdom to an even greater height, suggesting that aging can bring any older individual to a place of "gerotranscendence," where experience is less focused on time as a horizon and more on time as a moment. For Torstam, the wisdom of gerotranscendent individuals enables them to shed much of their fear of death as well as the human obsession with material things and superfluous social interactions. There is a sense of connection to a greater spirit in the universe and to the flow of generations past and yet to come. We could argue that this state actually represents a form of negative disengagement, but Torstam replies that such a view is culture-bound and ignores the positive aspects of gerotranscendence, which he equates with the supreme wisdom of old age.

Returning to the summer of 1972, I wonder how current politics would be transformed, for better or worse, if the surviving and now elderly players from that era returned to the scene, armed with all their wisdoms. McGovern has many ideas for what he would like to do, but he is content to leave it up to younger politicians, including his grandson, who recently ran for office in Milwaukee, Wisconsin, and lost. Perhaps there is still some hesitation on McGovern's part; he is, after all, the man who during the Vietnam War cried out on the Senate floor, "I'm fed up to the ears with old men dreaming up wars for young men to die in." If we ponder his admonition, we might ask whether it is natural and expected for the old to step aside and let the young assume the reins of power and decisionmaking. But perhaps the opposite is true—the aged should have a greater role because of their wisdom.

Any answer today is largely a thought experiment, because most elderly retire from both the workforce and positions of power in their mid- to late sixties—a relatively young point in the scheme of old age. But perhaps the vision of greater involvement of our elderly can at least be approximated. In 1997, for example, former South African president Nelson Mandela brought together a diverse group of prominent older world leaders for a unique forum. Could these illustrious, aged individuals serve as an influential, experienced, and independent group of peacebuilders to be called "the Elders"? Since the group's creation, several of these Elders have traveled around the globe to various sites of war and oppression, hoping to bring their collective wisdom to bear on seemingly intractable conflicts. Although their individual political bents might belie their independent labels, the existence of such a group puts to the test the questions of whether old age actually confers a unique, *wiser* perspective and whether such a perspective can be translated into action. Time may tell.

I have learned, then, that it is easy to puff up wisdom into a great force of history. But wisdom in its truest and most common form is not sitting in judgment like King Solomon or trotting the globe like the Elders to weigh the woes and conflicts of humankind. The individuals who manage such feats are few and far between. Instead, wisdom shines forth in the daily tumult of aging. And a day in the life of an elder may be like the Miami summer of 1972, where chaos and order and pageantry and protest coexisted, where hippies and politicians, radicals and Republicans, potheads and rabbis all came together in one hot, crowded, tear-gas-filled island to make a point about the future of the country. Wisdom serves to calm this maelstrom, providing a way of thinking, feeling, and experiencing that brings order, harmony, and, for many, a great measure of happiness.

Bereft

"You are no longer my son. I hate you."

The hand that penned these words is now a bony and blemished relic of a once powerful woman. I envision the actual pen as a heavyweight sterling silver Montblanc, befitting a woman of wealth and prestige who doted on her husband and his many interests. But there was neither dignity nor doting in this same woman's letter to a wayward son. Her searing words were scrawled on a piece of lined notepaper, with disjointed letters barely able to sit adjacent to each other. Whether it was true hate that motivated this woman's letter or merely the bewildered and reactive anger of a wounded mother cannot be known. It is clear, however, that the long-standing feud between this mother and her son eventually shattered the last vestiges of their relationship, and they parted ways permanently following the

death of her husband. She was bereft of all family and arrived
at our facility as if out of the ether, without penny or home.

In appearance Miriam was a stately woman, meticulously
groomed, her white hair pulled back in a tight bun. She described the central narrative in her life in bold terms: She came
from wealth and married into wealth, and her husband was a
successful banker and the love of her life. But her children were
"rotten thieves" who swindled her out of her personal fortune.
She denied any history of abuse or neglect of the children, nor
did she admit to any family trauma or other arguments. "I tried
to fix things up," she argued, "but my son demanded money in
order to visit me." That offense, she contended, prompted the
poison pen letter. From her arrival at the nursing home to my
first interview with her, Miriam had received no visitors and
had had no outside contacts. She occasionally spoke of distant
cousins who had lost track of her.

I have, unfortunately, seen many similarly bereft aged individuals. Some, like Miriam, are vicious in their descriptions
of absent children or family, whereas others exist quietly and
without protest, providing little or no explanation for their solitude. Occasionally, the person has a telltale history of substance
abuse, pathological gambling, chronic mania, personality disorder, or abusive behaviors that clearly drove family members
away. Other times the family members themselves suffer from
mental illness or are abusive or neglectful. In most cases these
older individuals appear friendly and cooperative, yet incredulous at their fate. There are almost always missing pieces to their
social and clinical histories that limit attempts to understand
them and prevent potential reconciliations. They arrive with so

many years of broken promises, lost fortunes, and burned bridges behind them that old age seems an unlikely time to heal.

Getting involved with these individuals raises its own challenges. Sometimes I learn from probing the histories of these lonely elders that they were, in fact, abusive or uncaring individuals. One daughter told me that when she was a child, her father used to dump cold buckets of water on her head for the smallest behavioral infraction. She will call to inquire about his health, but she will not see him. Another adult child hinted that her father was a sexual predator but could not bring herself to reveal more. She never visits. Sometimes these past behaviors are repeated in small ways, such as when Miriam accused her aides of being thieves who stole several pieces of costume jewelry that later appeared hidden in her room. With other bereft individuals, their appearances are so banal that it is hard to imagine why anyone would have abandoned them.

Knowing the history, however, may require some mental juggling. For instance, how does a mental health care provider form a therapeutic bond with a known sexual predator? Or a racist? How does a clinician feel empathy for a depressed patient who used to beat his children? It may be easier for an internist or a surgeon to face these patients, because their priority and duty are to heal the physical illness or injury at hand without having to probe the social history. The Hippocratic Oath of doctors tending to wounded enemy soldiers or terrorists during wartime does not discriminate on the basis of creed, even if it is a disturbing one. And in the rush of treatment, the doctor's ignorance of the patient's past sins may provide a protective emotional barrier.

The psychotherapeutic care of these older individuals is different, however, as it requires clinicians to learn about and understand past behaviors and their underlying causes. It might also require clinicians to subscribe to treatment goals that they reject in their hearts, such as helping an abuser to feel less depressed or to sleep better. The abandoning family members may resent or even obstruct attempts to help the patient, viewing clinicians as collaborators.

I recently began working on a family tree for my paternal relatives. As I called distant cousins around the country and slowly pieced each branch together, I began to feel a profound deepening of my own connections to both my father and his kin. I also saw how easily people could lose track of one another and how branches of the tree could break off and isolate individuals or families from one another. This experience led me to imagine Miriam as a small twig pruned from a tree, falling to the ground and being blown by the wind far from its trunk of origin.

Miriam, however, was wiser and more resourceful than I gave her credit. She became an integral part of the unit by befriending many other residents and staff. She was particular about whom she associated with, but bold nonetheless, and within several months had built up a social network throughout the nursing home. She had, in essence, formed a new family consisting of members who knew nothing or cared nothing about her past. This stance, I realize, is also essential when caring for most of these bereft older individuals. Regardless of past behaviors, they have arrived and must be tended to. I rarely know the exact truth of their past, and so I have to focus on their present and future. This is not an act of absolution but one of wisdom and adaptation, and serves as a necessary act of humanity in the final stages of life.

Just Words

What a loud voice cannot convey is better carried by a whistle across the deep valleys, or barrancos, of La Gomera, a small mountainous island in the Canary Island chain off the coast of West Africa. Over centuries the shepherds of La Gomera developed a unique way to shape these whistles into an actual language, called Silbo Gomero. To untrained ears, these whistles strike the brain like any other nonsensical sounds, perceived but meaningless. To speakers of Silbo, however, these whistled communications activate the same parts of the brain involved in language comprehension and expression.

One lesson here is that a language can consist of something more than just words, be it whistles, tongue clicks, or hand gestures. This lesson is learned the hard way by older individuals with severe language disturbances, called aphasia, who struggle to find an elusive language without words that will override their jumbled linguistic circuits. In the beginning, however, this "language of one" is nonsensical because, according to the philosopher Ludwig Wittgenstein, the true meaning of a language emerges through its use among people. But with time and interaction, a new form of communication may emerge.

My older patient Rachel had once been fluent in five languages—not an uncommon skill for individuals born and raised along many European frontiers prior to World War II. At the time of our first meeting, however, the speech of this elderly polyglot had been reduced to a nonfluent cadence of chopped words that resembled some English and at least some Hungarian. As long as she didn't speak, however, she had an air of normality. I often bumped into her strolling along the brick footpaths near the assisted living facility in which she lived. She always remembered me and would greet me with a kiss on my hand and a sincere embrace.

I initially suspected that Rachel suffered from a relatively rare form of dementia afflicting the frontal and temporal lobes of her brain because her symptoms seemed to consist solely of impaired language function, including difficulty expressing words and an inability to name things. Her brain scan was unremarkable, and her medical history, physical exam, and labs were unrevealing. She refused to sit for neuropsychological testing. With time came worsening language function, behavioral outbursts, and more cognitive decline, still suggesting the rare form of dementia I initially suspected but also the more common Alzheimer's disease.

More pressing than her diagnosis, however, was the question of how best to communicate with Rachel. Once she came to the clinic in great distress, crying out unintelligibly and grimacing whenever her abdomen was touched. Her condition seemed clinically to be some form of gastrointestinal illness, and yet an extensive workup that included an abdominal X-ray, CAT scan, ultrasound, and, eventually, a colonoscopy was unrevealing. Rachel returned from the hospital calmer, but with the lingering mystery of what she had been trying to tell us.

There are many debates about the difference between words and deeds. Lofty words may invoke great power, but words not backed up by deeds may be ultimately meaningless. A student of Wittgenstein might argue, however, that because reality stems from the shared logic and meaning of our language, words *are* deeds. Anything that lies beyond the logic of our speech is otherwise meaningless, worthy only of silence. And yet I have sometimes found that the patients who speak the loudest are those in whom language has dissolved. Like the shepherds of La Gomera, they are forced by necessity to shape words into whistles.

The key question is whether these whistles—in whatever form they manifest—will hit the brains of listeners as nonsensical sounds or as meaningful expressions. I am reminded of the legend of King Solomon, who was said to have understood the language of the birds, and I ask, "Who among us has the patience and wisdom to listen closely and try to understand the whistling and warbling of our own linguistically impaired elderly?"

I came close to this ideal state one day when Rachel burst into my office, grabbed me by the arm, pulled me out of my chair, and without making a sound escorted me arm in arm down the hallway of the clinic. Several nurses watched the scene incredulously and followed behind, wondering whether Rachel had gone mad. As we rounded the corner and entered one of the bays off the hallway, Rachel pushed me up to her sister-in-law, Emma, who was sitting in a wheelchair. She gestured at Emma and let out a high-pitched whine saturated with a pained inflection. The sound made me wince, and I instinctively knew that Emma needed help. Indeed, Emma had been trying to call the doctor, and none had appeared. Rachel had felt her pain and was able to convey it to me.

Emma looked at me and raised her arms upward: "God has forgotten me," she sighed. I surveyed the scene in front of her, now surrounded by a retinue of interested and concerned staff members, with Rachel standing by, beaming proudly. In the moment, I understood Rachel perfectly. I turned to Emma. "Has God forgotten you?" I asked, and then answered, "I don't think so."

Liar, Liar

"Lies, my dear boy, are found out immediately,
because they are of two sorts. There are lies that
have short legs, and lies that have long noses."

—CARLO COLLODI, PINOCCHIO

This was a long-nosed lie, and I knew that payback was coming. Several minutes earlier Ginny had bulldozed into my office with her walker. "Why the hell am I here? What's this all about?" I stared at her for a moment in silence. "All I want from you is my scooter!" she demanded. "Give it back!" The bare truth was that Ginny was moderately demented and perpetually hostile and paranoid. I was getting calls from nursing staff telling me that she had fixated on one particular chair on her unit and was forbidding anyone else to sit in it. It had even come to blows one day when she punched poor Victor, who had unknowingly sat in "her" chair, his deaf ears not hearing her stomping and curses from behind.

Fueling her anger was the fact that for several months Ginny had been demanding the return of her electric scooter. The nursing home administrator and I had recently made a decision to restrict her from using it for safety reasons, and I was supposed to inform her that day. However, given her demeanor and her hatred of psychiatrists, I feared an explosion.

"I'm one of your doctors," I stated, intentionally leaving out my specialty. She fired back, "Can I have my scooter?" I hesitated to answer. "Well, Ginny, we haven't yet decided," I lied. Ginny's angry face seemed to scrunch up into a single point that jabbed at the fragile bubble of my lie. She could be amazingly prescient even in the fog of dementia and paranoia. "Liar! Liar!" she accused, and then stood up and shrieked at me, "Go to hell!" I quickly opened the door and let her pass. I could hear her carrying on as she traversed the long hallway of the clinic. "That doctor can go to hell!" she called out repeatedly, her words echoing back to my office several times. "He can go to hell!" In her wrath she seemed to stretch my long-nosed lie past each office bay, around the front desk, and out into the courtyard in front of the clinic. Maybe it would have been better if I had simply told the truth.

Truthfulness is the foundation of the doctor-patient relationship, both as a method of discourse and as one of the "most widely praised character traits" of a doctor. Gone are the days when doctors withheld certain diagnoses or treatment details from patients. If anything, doctors today are often forced to disclose excess and sometimes unnecessary information due to concerns about liability or to patients who have already canvassed the Internet on their own and have pressing questions. The doctor's challenge is to present what he or she knows to be true about the diagnosis and its treatment options and to do so in a manner that truly informs the patient. But there are limitations and pitfalls to this process, as illustrated in the following paraphrased conversation I recently had with a seventy-five-year-old moderately demented patient and his wife:

> PATIENT: Doctor, I know I can still drive. Just let me take a test.
>
> DOCTOR A: I'm sorry, Mr. K, but I can't help you with that. As we discussed, your memory impairment makes it unsafe for you to drive.
>
> PATIENT: Just let me take the test. I can drive just fine.
>
> DOCTOR A: The memory testing tells us that you would not be a safe driver.
>
> PATIENT: My memory is not that bad. I know I can drive.
>
> PATIENT'S WIFE: Honey, I told you that the car is not working now and needs to be fixed. Let's talk about it later.
>
> PATIENT: Okay.

Mr. K's wife did what caregivers for individuals with dementia often do—she placated his concerns for the moment and then redirected him, in essence telling a lie. Should doctors ever do the same thing?

According to a leading book on medical ethics, "Careful management of medical information—including nondisclosure, deception, and lying—will all occasionally be justified when veracity conflicts with other obligations." Every clinician has encountered situations in which being too bluntly honest about a diagnosis can actually be harmful to the patient, and so we employ what is euphemistically referred to as "benevolent deception." Consider mentally fragile patients with whom full disclosure of a devastating diagnosis may cause excessive anxiety, abandonment of ongoing therapies, or total loss of hope. In these circumstances, strict adherence to the clinical virtues of truthfulness and candor risks violation of the core ethical principle to do no harm. We are left telling a series of what I term "short-legged lies," or partial truths that take small steps toward eventual and necessary disclosure of the complete truth.

As much as I urge eventual, complete disclosure of the truth to every patient, there are individuals with dementia who will not be able to appreciate the meaning of what they are told and cannot correctly distinguish between truth and deception. Perhaps there is still an obligation to at least go through the motions. I think about how I endeavor to always formally introduce myself to patients regardless of their mental state—even when they seem completely insensible. There is a transcendent ethical principle at stake here applying specifically to severely demented individuals: the preservation of their human dignity, even when they lack the ability to perceive its personal value. Truth-telling, in some form, appears to be a key part of this principle.

In work with cognitively impaired patients, there is a certain savoir faire to telling the truth, or a piece of it, without causing unnecessary confusion or anguish. "Frank but not blunt" is how one textbook characterizes the ideal approach, recommending that the clinician present the reality of a medical situation without causing the patient to lose all hope. This is a difficult and sometimes impossible tightrope to walk, especially when a clinician has to convey a diagnosis in which there is no hope for cure. In those moments clergy are often more skilled than doctors at providing hope for something other than physical redemption.

I recently had to inform a relatively young couple in their late fifties of a diagnosis of Alzheimer's disease in the husband. There was no escaping a frank presentation of the data and the logical conclusion. I was girded with the knowledge of a recent study suggesting that, contrary to the fears of many doctors, patients are unlikely to demonstrate catastrophic reactions when a diagnosis of dementia is relayed. In fact, many are relieved. In this case, however, there was no visible relief. Instead, I saw the color drain out of the woman's face as the meaning of the diagnosis settled in. Her tense facial expression relaxed, no longer anticipating the verdict, but then began to absorb the tears tracing a growing look of despair. She had many questions that I knew would come in time, but I wasn't ready to lay out any more truths that day. It was not even the moment to talk of hope—of medications, therapeutic programs, and research. It was a moment instead to retreat into the practice of medicine described by the poet Virgil as *ars muta*, the "silent art." Bioethicist James F. Drane captures a more modern-day description of this form of truth-telling: "There are times for both the patient and the doctor when silence both carries deep meaning and is an appropriate expression of truth."

Rules of Four

"His head feels like a furry leaf, but softer."

This was the unintentional poetry of a six-year-old boy meeting his newborn brother for the first time. That "furry leaf" is now a wild bush of brown curls that sails through the house, jumping from couch to chair and through clutters of overturned toys, Legos, and puzzle pieces with the energy that only a four-year-old boy can expend. I am tired just watching him. I think to myself how the universe of a four-year-old has its own rules. He lives in the moment. He speaks what is on his mind. Sometimes he asks for what he wants; sometimes he screams for it. Regardless, I love every hair on his head. No matter what he does or how he looks, he is always beloved to me. And aside from the few instances in which he tells me that I'm "fired," I know that he feels the same. These guiding principles for my

four-year-old son and me—or "rules of four," as I call them—
are a binding force between us.

On many nights I engage in a ritual familiar to most parents
and steal silently into his room just to watch him breathe. I sit
next to his bed and lay my head on his pillow, my nose nestled
into curls that smell of oatmeal and honey from his bath. The
only sounds are his soft rhythmic breaths and the hushed blow-
ing of the air conditioner. His expression is serene. It is in these
quiet moments that I sometimes pose questions that perhaps
only a geriatrician would consider: Who will attend to this precious child when he is ninety? Who will guard him as he sleeps,
guide him while awake, and treasure him merely for his presence?
There will come a time, I imagine, a time long in the future,
when my youngest son will be an old man, bereft of his parents
and siblings. Who will love him and care for him like we do?

There have been many evenings when I have walked the
halls of the nursing home in which I work, attending to last-
minute orders or residents' needs. I often stop to look at the
photographs that family members have posted in the clear plastic
shadow boxes outside many of the rooms. Black-and-white
photographs of ancient childhood scenes mingle with formal
wedding poses, soldiers in crisp uniforms, beloved pets, and
color shots of children and grandchildren. Outside one room a
twenty-five-year-old model strikes a pose in a stylish black dress
with arm-length gloves, her fingers balancing an ivory cigarette
holder in her lips. Inside the room, the frail body of this same
woman, now eighty-five years old, lies silently in her bed. Outside another room I see an entire lifetime before me: an infant
child in his mother's arms, a World War II marine, a father with

children, and then a retiree sitting with his grandchildren. With one eye I regard this circle of life; with the other I peer into his room where he sits asleep in a wheelchair. And I wonder, To whom are these residents still beloved?

Rule #1: When you need something, ask. When you don't get it, scream.

Anita reminded me of this rule the other day. I sat with her in my office, thumbing through her chart and reading—*again*—that she was screaming at staff. There were a few choice words that she preferred to use to get what she needed, and they seemed to work, although at a cost. Her undergarments were clean, but she was not well liked. "Anita," I said calmly. "*Anita*," I repeated with a little more emphasis, and implored, "You cannot scream at the nurses." My face was serious, but I softened it with a half-smile, mouth closed. We had talked about this before, but I still wanted to be patient with her. "Listen, Dr. Agronin," she said, "you don't understand what *I* do, and *I* am a pro at this. If I don't scream, they won't come to help me."

Anita stared me down, and I wasn't sure what to say. I know how things work on a busy floor in a nursing home. The staff work hard, and they cannot drop everything and run instantly each time a resident rings the call bell. Sometimes screaming does work better than softness. "Remember rule number one," I thought. Anita lives in the moment. She is mildly cognitively impaired and majorly impetuous. At eighty-eight years old, confined to a wheelchair, widowed, and racked with pain from a large sore on her behind, she has lost all manner of discretion. She tells it like it is, and if a bowel movement is pressing and she needs help, you'll know it. Here is my disclaimer: I do not endorse or condone this approach in the nursing home; in fact, it is my job to treat it. But I do understand it.

Rule #2: Every hair on your head is important to me.

If you think about how precious young children are to their parents, no one is surprised when they dote over them, marveling at every word and each new hair and tooth. Then why are we so surprised when older family members do essentially the same thing? Edgar was one such son who baffled and annoyed the nursing home staff. He used to measure his ninety-five-year-old mother's temperature to the tenth of a degree, trusting neither the thermometer at the nurse's station nor the judgment of the medical staff. According to the doctors, normal body temperature is 98.6 degrees Fahrenheit, with some variation by time of day and method of measurement. According to Edgar, the normal body temperature range for his mother was between 97 and 98.2 degrees Fahrenheit; anything above was, by his empirical method, a fever that required workup. He kept a log by her bedside with his own daily measurements.

I was called one day to mediate a dispute between Edgar and his mother's doctor. For two days Edgar had recorded a temperature of 98.8 degrees, and he was panicked. He demanded a chest X-ray for his mother, along with urine, sputum, and blood cultures. The doctor refused, stating that 98.8 degrees was not a fever and that there was no evidence of infection. Edgar threatened to report the facility to the state. I pulled the doctor aside, knowing that trying to negotiate with Edgar was futile; he was worked up into such a lather that my very presence as a psychiatrist might put him over the edge. "I know that he can be unreasonable," I admitted, "and I know that he has an obsessive-compulsive personality dis—"

"Yeh think?" the doctor interrupted me. "I'm drawing a line in the sand here."

"Don't do that," I suggested, trying to reason with her without taking Edgar's side. "She has a little bit of a cough—will a chest X-ray hurt anyone? In the very least it will get him off of your back."

The X-ray was taken, and it showed, to everyone's surprise, except Edgar's, a rip-roaring pneumonia. If the doctor had waited one more day, Edgar's mother might have ended up in the hospital. Rule number two came to mind: It's not her hair but every tenth of a degree in her body temperature that is important to Edgar. He knows her and cares for her more than anyone else ever will. His observations and demands may be a burden for the doctors and staff and may challenge their clinical judgment, but they stem from a fierce sense of love and protection.

Rule #3: No matter how you look, you are adorable to me.

Jorge was in love with Marta, deeply in love. After forty years of marriage and five children, the fire might be expected to burn a little lower. The love I see in many similar couples is warm, reserved, and practical, like the glowing embers of a small fire. For Jorge, his love for Marta was like a burning torch. His request to me, then, was not surprising; "Do anything to bring her back." Marta had suffered a massive stroke several months earlier but remained in a coma. The only thing keeping her alive was the ventilator next to the bed, pumping oxygen through the ribbed blue tubing hooked into the tracheotomy site in her neck. After lingering in the hospital for several weeks, she had been transferred to our long-term vent unit.

Marta was motionless in the bed, showing an occasional flutter of her eyelids that Jorge interpreted as some form of communication. The scene in the room was intimidating to most visitors. On one side of the bed hung a bag of beige liquid nutrients being infused into Marta's stomach through a soft gray tube. Adjacent to the bed a urine bag was hanging visibly from the metal side rails. In the background was the constant, rhythmic whoosh of the ventilator. The room felt humid and had an antiseptic smell. On most days I found Jorge hovering at her side, smoothing her hair and saying, "You are beautiful, *mi amor*." Here was a vision of rule number three: the personage of Marta, lying insensibly in bed with a full diaper and the odors of bodily fluids, surrounded by tubes and machines and pumps—but still adorable to her true love.

I had spoken to the pulmonologist about Jorge's request to try a cocktail of stimulants to bring Marta out of her vegetative state, but she was hesitant. Marta's cardiac status was fragile, and multiple brain scans and neurological exams had confirmed irreversible brain damage. We could still care for her body, but her mind had slipped too far away. Nevertheless, Jorge's torch was undimmed.

Rule #4: No matter what you do, I still love you.

I do not understand how Bonnie manages to care for her mother, Shelly, at home. Shelly is morbidly obese, confined to a wheelchair, moderately demented, and *mean*. She doesn't ask for things; she screams once, curses, and then tries to pinch or bite if she isn't tended to immediately. She wakes Bonnie up at night for no specific reason, yelling for her daughter to come to her mother's room. I have tried everything to calm Shelly, but with each new medication trial comes a new side effect: confusion, agitation, tremors, and diarrhea. Ironically, the only medication that has worked, and that she has tolerated, is Thorazine. For most of my patients, Thorazine would be the equivalent of a chemical sledgehammer, so I never use it. Even so, it merely slows Shelly down without stopping her rampages.

At our last meeting Shelly was relatively calm. She denied her behaviors, insisting that her daughter was lying to me. I contrasted the descriptions of Shelly's behavior with her beautifully dressed and manicured appearance in my office. "What did you do in the past?" I asked her. Her remote memory was still intact, and she described to me her life as a young model, actress, and singer. "It's true," Bonnie told me, gazing at her mother lovingly; "you were quite a singer, sweetie." Shelly basked in the love for a moment and then shot back, "You're my sister, aren't you?" Bonnie didn't miss a beat: "No, remember sweetie, I'm your daughter, Bonnie." Shelly was not convinced. In fact, she looked disgusted.

As I listened to a litany of problem behaviors, I looked straight at Shelly. She smiled knowingly and then confessed, "Since I don't have a mother to give me attention, I *have* to behave that way." This was a moment of lucidity and honesty, and it faded quickly. But I understood: rule number one crossed with rule number four. Shelly wanted her mother, and so did Bonnie.

These rules of four represent for me the bond between parent and child, and I have learned that they do not stop at the age of four. The child may now be sixty and the parent eight-five, but the rules still apply. Some rules change with the person or context, whereas others are inviolable. I see this all the time in the nursing home, although now the roles of parent and child have been reversed. Sometimes it is an older spouse or sibling, or a niece or nephew, who fills in the dyad. As a doctor, I am sometimes surprised by how emotional or irrational these caregivers can become. But I have to catch myself at those moments, examine the relationship, and remember the rules. If I can empathize with their own rules of four or five or *eighty-five,* then I can intervene in a caring way. And my sincerest hope is that if my own precious child is the one lying in a nursing home bed someday long in the future, with my caring hand only a memory, that someone else's protective wing will be there—and let it be as emotional or irrational as is required to care for him.

Part V
A Million Sparks

Seeing, in April, hostas unfurl like arias,

and tulips, white cups inscribed with licks of flame,

gaze feverish, grown almost to my waist,

and the oak raise new leaves for benediction,

I mourn for what does not come back: the movie theater—

reels spinning out vampire bats, last trains,

the arc of Chaplin's cane, the hidden doorways—

struck down for a fast-food store; your rangy stride;

my shawl of hair; my mother's grand piano.

My mother.

How to make it new,

how to find the gain in it? Ask the sea

at sunrise how a million sparks can fly

over dead bones.

—GRACE SCHULMAN, "CELEBRATION"

Final Acts

Old age is the closing act of life, as of a drama, and we ought to leave when the play grows wearisome, especially if we have had our fill.

—Marcus Cicero, "On Old Age"

Here is a scene from the final act of a man's life: A small crowd of spectators, all clad in blue and white scrubs, were gathered around the imposing figure of an eighty-five-year-old hospital patient. His outstretched arm jabbed toward the crowd while the other cradled the soiled bedsheet wrapped around his body like a toga. "Hear me! Hear me!" he bellowed at each staff member, his face wide-eyed and contorted like a crazed orator. With each shout he spun a quarter-turn from his perch on the floor, spreading out the pool of urine in which he sat. Each nurse tried, in turn, to entreat the man to calm down and return to his room. Thirty minutes into his increasing agitation, I received a phone call requesting an urgent psychiatric consultation. I entered the scene and asked that the crowd disperse, save one kindly nurse. After a few minutes without an audience, the man calmed down and was coaxed into a wheelchair.

Scene two occurred a day later and opened with this same man lying in a hospital bed. He was again agitated, begging for someone to hear him but unable to make his needs known. I prescribed a mild sedative to calm him, but with little effect. He languished for several days with spreading infection and delirium, insensible to surrounding family, and then he passed away. This short drama was all that I witnessed of the man's long life. I was one of his doctors only at the end, and I missed the last few years of kidney failure, chronic pain, and dementia. Prior to that, he had been a successful architect, an avid traveler and photographer, and the patriarch of a large family. In reflecting back on all of the pain, indignity, confusion, and agitation of his last few years, the man's son raised a logical question: "What's the point? If that is old age," he wondered, "who needs it?"

This is a common question today and has been a common question since antiquity. Indeed, the search for answers that provide some meaning to aging is an ancient pursuit, explored in depth in the Bible and in later writings by major Greek and Roman philosophers. "Rise up before the aged, and honor the face of the sage," instructs Leviticus 19:32. From the vantage point of the Bible, this is an easy task because most of the major players, from Adam to Noah and from Abraham and Sarah to Moses, remained active and influential in later life. They served as role models for aging and countered darker voices, such as are found in Job 12:1, where the reader is warned to remember days of youth, "Before the evil days come, And the years draw nigh, when thou shalt say: 'I have no pleasure in them.'"

Ancient Greek philosophy was less sanguine about aging. According to the hedonistic teachings of Aristippus of Cyrene (435–356 BC), the pursuit of pleasure was the supreme good, especially the immediate gratifications obtained by the body. The later writings of Epicurus (342–270 BC) focused less on physical pleasure and more on the measured pursuit of mental tranquility, coupled with the absence of fear and physical pain. For both schools of thought, old age presented a serious challenge because illness, pain, and infirmity often limited the pursuit of most forms of pleasure. In essence, aging was equated with death. This is not surprising given that the average life expectancy in ancient Rome was twenty-eight years.

But today the average lifespan is now close to eighty. In our deepest aspirations we hope for a *good* old age, a *golden* age where gold means a time of interpersonal richness, wisdom, and gilded reflection on the deeds of our lives. But although we can extol the sense of integrity and satisfaction that can come with a life lived long and well, we must ask what would be the meaning and value in aging for those who have failed to achieve this? In 44 BC Roman philosopher and statesman Cicero wrote in his essay "On Old Age" that "old age is respectable as long as it asserts itself, maintains it rights, is subservient to no one." If this is true, then what do we make of those aged individuals who can no longer assert themselves or who are dependent on caregivers for satisfying most of their needs? Cicero himself seemed to recognize a point of no return: "As the pursuits of the earlier

periods fall away, so do those of old age, and when this happens
weariness of life brings a season ripe for death."

A time for death? I call this the "enough is enough" argument, and I have heard it from countless older individuals in
the throes of illness. I have also heard it from baby boomers ob-
sessed with their independence and right to make all health care
decisions as they project themselves into an imagined state of
dementia and disability. Philosophers and ethicists have a version
called the "fair innings argument," which postulates that those
aged individuals who have already experienced many good years
of life should not be endlessly preserved at the expense of
younger individuals. This argument is pursued in the writings
of medical ethicist Daniel Callahan, who raises concerns about
the disproportionate amount of resources spent on extending
the length but not necessarily the quality of the lives of older
individuals. He asks whether "there is an obligation to keep the
elderly alive as long as possible, regardless of the cost of doing
so." Perhaps, he asserts, "there is a duty to help young people
to become old people, but not to help the old become still older
indefinitely." And how does Callahan define "old"? "My own
answer," he states, "is that someone is old when it can be said
that he or she has had a 'full life,' by which I mean enough time
to do most (though not necessarily all) of the things that a life
makes possible: education, family, work, and so on." Callahan
imagines that between the ages of seventy-five and eighty most
people have lived a full life, and he then suggests that most of
us would not regard death at that time as a tragedy.

This is a well-crafted argument from a thousand feet high,
but it often flounders on the ground in face-to-face interactions

with older people. It may also lead to cynical and fatalistic attitudes toward both medical care and meaningful activities for the oldest and most debilitated individuals. The "what's the point?" argument engenders apathy and resignation among younger generations who could be vitally involved with their elders. It also prompts the great fear that limiting resources to the aged leads down a slippery slope toward a society like the fictional Republic of Britanura envisioned by novelist Anthony Trollope in his 1882 work *The Fixed Period*. In Britanura the "problems" of old age are solved by mandatory suicide at the age of sixty-eight. The 1967 novel *Logan's Run* is a modern version of Trollope's dystopia, as is the world in the 1973 movie *Soylent Green*, in which older individuals are gently euthanized and then turned into food.

This latter argument is exaggerated, of course, because no one would argue for such a world. But in the hinterlands of the aged, in quiet rooms where the oldest of the old dwell, there are raging arguments about what to do about aging, sometimes solved by passive or active unsanctioned neglect. And in many cases even our best intentions seem futile and they utterly fail, pushed aside by what I call the "Four Horsemen of Old Age": depression, dementia, delirium, and destitution. In nearly every tragic case of aging, one or more of these reapers are in attendance. And when they hold the mind in their grip of dissolution, any talk of potential quality of life seems comical. We pity and sometimes shake our heads at caregivers who persist in loving and attending to diseased or dying older loved ones or who rage at their attendants in hope of salvaging some last vestige of a good old age.

I have a deep and enduring fascination and affection for these aged souls. Their care is my life's work and my passion. But many of the countless older patients whom I have treated have tested me as a doctor, and I have sometimes failed. And they have forced me to admit that old age is not always what I want it to be. Thus, the sentiments behind Cicero's resignation and Mr. K's son's despair are understandable. At this point, the doctor reaches the limits of all knowledge and technique. Cicero seems to rule the day only as long as the aged mind is intact and the body is still able to secure its basic needs; after that, many elders reasonably assert, "Close the curtain. Enough is enough!"

I have seen, however, how sparks of humanity persist until the final moments, and I must state, "Perhaps we are missing something." Even without mental rationality, there are perception, emotion, and imagination. Even without the ability to walk or even move independently, there are still movement and sensation. Even for Mr. K., there were years of existence prior to his final moments that were filled with the potential for meaningful experiences. We cannot reverse death, but dementia, depression, delirium, and destitution are challenges we *can* do something about. If Cicero had the audacity to challenge both the hedonism and the ageism of Roman culture, why can't we push our own cultural envelope a bit further? Here the young can help the old to form intergenerational connections, create vital activities, relieve pain and mental suffering, and ensure a dignified existence. Cicero, too, recognized these timeless responsibilities: "When the end comes what has passed has flowed away, and all that is left is what you have achieved by virtue and good deeds." In the final act, it is not life that fails our efforts, but our lack of effort that fails the still pulsating life.

I contrast the last stage of life and its profound challenges to a vantage point one step beyond the passing of an individual. My friend Eli is a volunteer member of a *chevra kadisha*, or Jewish burial society, in which he helps to ritually prepare bodies for burial in what is known as the *tahara* ritual. This responsibility is considered one of the holiest acts in Judaism, because the deceased can never thank those who accord this final act of respect. As Eli has described to me, the ritual cleansing, washing, and enshrouding of the body are performed in a careful and dignified manner and are accompanied by the recitation of specific prayers. The four volunteers do not converse during the ceremony other than required, and they never turn their backs to the body or expose it in an undignified manner. It is a wholly anonymous task, without any thanks given or received. The holiness of the act is thanks enough.

The respect accorded to the deceased is not unique to Judaism but is enshrined and ritualized in most religious and secular burial rites. In general, both the ritual and ethics of death are well structured in our society, focusing on values of respect and dignity for the deceased and comfort and meaning for their mourners. With many older individuals, however, the final months and years of life are often folded together and considered a living death, but never given the amount of attention, ritual, or respect accorded when death finally arrives. For if we regard every second of life as precious, then the incredible degree of respect that we naturally accord to the deceased must also be extended to the living. Hospice for the dying must be preceded by a movement of meaning and vitality for the still living! Otherwise, we end up missing profound opportunities to understand our elders and, by extension, ourselves. We also miss opportunities to encourage and gather together the still present sparks of life that can transform the experience of aging into a more positive and meaningful time. My older patients have shown me what can be.

Mended

According to legend, when the Angel of Death descends to earth to take a soul from the world of the living, he stands at the head of the dying one's bed and draws the sword from his sheath, preparing for the final moment. But Aaron the peacemaker, brother of Moses, was spared this act due to his righteousness. God himself kissed Aaron's soul and brought it to heaven.

�֍✖✖

As my patient Aron lay in his hospital bed, he had a strange vision. A figure emerged from the darkness and penetrated the curtain around his bed, hovering over his face and poised to strike. Despite his physical debility, Aron gathered up his strength and swung his fist at the shadowy intruder, wrestling with it before knocking it away. He awoke the next morning and was wheeled into surgery.

A month before I met Aron, the circumstances of our meeting were set in motion. As I was preparing for a trip to Boston, my assistant brought me a message from Aron's daughter-in-law begging me to see him for a second opinion. She explained that he was an eighty-four-year-old survivor of Auschwitz who had recently been diagnosed with Alzheimer's disease and was deteriorating rapidly. Although she had already learned that my clinic did not accept Aron's health insurance, she inquired whether I could still see him the following week when her husband would be in South Florida and could bring him to an appointment. Although the urgency of the consult was not clear to me, I agreed to see Aron on my return.

My trip to Boston turned out to be quite prescient of the coming events with Aron. After a nearly fourteen-year absence, I was returning to the site of my residency training in psychiatry to deliver a lecture on the topic of late-life personality development. McLean Hospital was one of America's first major asylums for the mentally ill, designed in the 1800s when a serene, park-like atmosphere was considered a mainstay of psychiatric care. Seeing the familiar panorama of rolling hills, grand oak trees, and Gothic brick buildings on campus brought back strong memories, even though I assumed that much had changed in the many years I had been away. My trip felt like a homecoming as I encountered so many of the same colleagues with whom I had worked years before—even several supervisors whom I had imagined were long retired. Appearances had changed a bit but not spirits, and I was exhilarated by the visit.

In my lecture I spoke about how, although personality seemed cast in stone early in life, there remained the great potential for positive change over time, for adaptation and even rejuvenation in the face of late-life stresses. In clinical work with the elderly, however, there is the risk of getting accustomed to the opposite: viewing constant decline as fate and restoration of the past as fantasy. As it turned out, my encounter with Aron illustrated the potentially disastrous consequences of such an attitude.

Aron arrived for his appointment late on a Friday afternoon, accompanied by his oldest son. I was immediately concerned when I saw how slowly he shuffled into my office, as if he were wearing heavy shoes magnetically stuck to the floor. He had a baffled expression on his face and could barely speak except for a few phrases in a mix of English, Hebrew, and Yiddish. His son reported that Aron lived alone in a small retirement community near Ft. Lauderdale, where he had been quite active with the large group of Holocaust survivors. Amazingly, he also reported that only four months ago Aron had been driving a car and functioning independently. The family was deeply concerned about this precipitous change in his function, and they were furious with his primary care physician, who had refused to authorize a brain scan because he reasoned that it would not change the diagnosis or management of Alzheimer's disease. Instead, he had sent Aron to a psychiatrist, who diagnosed depression and started him on an antidepressant medication.

In truth, it took only a few moments for me to realize that the clinical picture looked nothing like Alzheimer's disease but instead suggested a rapidly progressing neurological disorder that warranted immediate attention. Strokes can certainly cause the gait impairment seen with Aron, even when the actual event goes initially unrecognized. In some individuals, a variety of causes, including high blood pressure and diabetes, can cause tiny strokes in the lower regions of the brain. The silent, slow accumulation of these small areas of dead brain tissue eventually hits a tipping point where symptoms appear, often consisting of short-term memory loss, a slowing of movement and thought, and a propensity to apathy and depression. Aron's slowed gait fit this clinical picture, but his language dysfunction did not. A stroke large enough to cause his impaired speech would certainly have caused other, more devastating symptoms, which I did not detect.

Another possibility was a relatively uncommon but frequently misdiagnosed condition called normal pressure hydrocephalus, or NPH, in which the natural circulation of cerebrospinal fluid is disturbed, resulting in swelling of the inner chambers of the brain and compression of the surrounding tissue. To the doctor's eye, NPH produces a classic symptomatic triad of progressive dementia, gait disturbance, and urinary incontinence. The gait disturbance looks very much like Aron's walk, with each plodding step appearing to be strenuously resisting a strong magnetic pull to the ground. Although I certainly suspected NPH, Aron's language impairment was not consistent with its clinical picture.

Aron came to me with a diagnosis of Alzheimer's disease, but that is a slowly progressive disease of the brain where change unfolds over many years, not in just a few short months. Something else was going on with Aron that only a brain scan could show. Unfortunately, neither time nor Aron's insurance was in his favor at that moment. It was late on a Friday afternoon, and only his assigned physician could authorize the insurance company to approve a scan. I called repeatedly but did not hear back from the doctor. As Aron and his son waited, I tried repeatedly to make progress with the insurance, running a gauntlet of phone numbers and various departments, none of which took responsibility for the decision. Finally, I managed to reach a supervisor. I explained the dilemma and suggested—almost threatened—that without authorization for a brain scan I would be forced to send Aron to the emergency room at much greater cost. The supervisor relented, and within minutes I had Aron and his son out the door and on their way to our imaging facility. I went so far as to walk them out to their car and program the GPS to make certain that they made it to the facility before it closed for the day. The son called me a half hour later; they were there, but questions about whether Aron had a metal stent in his body would delay the scan for a day.

The next morning I received a phone call from the radiologist about an hour after the scan. I had never gotten such an urgent call from him before, and so I immediately suspected trouble. In fact, the news was ominous. He informed me that Aron had a huge cyst in his left frontal lobe with an associated tumor that was causing his entire brain to shift two centimeters away from its midline. The clinical symptoms now made perfect sense, because the large mass was pressing on both his brain's language center and a strip of brain tissue that controlled movement.

I reached Aron's sons to give them the news, and they were concerned but not surprised. We agreed that a neurosurgical consult was needed, and I called the primary care physician to get the ball rolling.

"Oh, yes, I know Aron," the doctor said; "he has Alzheimer's disease." "No," I countered, "he has a massive tumor in his skull." There was silence for a moment. I explained to him the findings from the brain scan and asked what the next step should be. The doctor instructed me to have Aron call his office Monday morning to schedule an appointment. Now I was angry and almost ready myself to drive Aron down to the nearest hospital. If he had been my own grandfather, I would have demanded faster action and moved heaven and earth to get it. I sought advice from a former college roommate who is now a neurosurgeon in Seattle. The news was not good, he cautioned, because such brain tumors in eighty-four-year-olds are often malignant, and without rapid treatment, Aron would soon die. Given the grim prognosis, I did not expect to see Aron again.

It took several days to get Aron to a neurosurgeon, and approximately ten days after our initial meeting he was admitted to the hospital for brain surgery that would attempt to drain the cyst and cut out as much of the adjacent tumor as possible. Although his vision of an unknown, shadowy visitor to his hospital bed the night before surgery seemed ominous, Aron interpreted it quite differently, feeling emboldened by his strength and confident that he had vanquished the intruder. As it turned out, the cyst was drained easily and the tumor was cut out completely from its perch on top of his brain. It was a completely benign growth, and Aron was cured.

Three weeks after surgery Aron himself drove to my office with his two sons as passengers in the car. "He's a little fast on the pedal," one son commented, "but that's nothing new." Aron strode into my office with a steady, *normal* gait. He threw his arms around me and hugged me, thanking me with tears in his eyes. In perfect, fluent English he told me about his desire to resume his previous independent life, despite his sons' concerns. I was so impressed that I invited him to sit and talk for an hour while I recorded his life history. Aron described his life in great detail, including his survival in Auschwitz, where he managed to fool his Nazi overseers during forced labor by rubbing charcoal on his face so that he looked as if he were working a lot harder than he actually was. And now, I thought, he had survived again by tricking fate. Recounting his experiences during the Holocaust certainly brought great sorrow to Aron, but that day he was stitched up a bit, temporarily mended by the opportunity to share an epic, defining story in his life that spoke of his bravery and faith in the face of certain doom. And in the listening, I felt a little mended myself, both amazed at his recovery and thrilled to see my elderly patient returned to a former state of function after nearly dying.

Nevertheless, I wondered deeply about Aron's presurgical vision of the shadowy intruder. Perhaps he had been hallucinating from the effects of the tumor or from the steroids prescribed to shrink the swelling in his brain. Perhaps the nurses had given him a sleeping pill that induced a mild delirium. Or perhaps the silent visitor wasn't the Angel of Death but was Raphael, the Angel of Healing, who once visited Abraham the patriarch and healed the wounds of his circumcision as a reward for his profound faith in God. I imagined that this visitor lay atop Aron like the prophet Elisha, who resurrected the dead child of the Shunammite woman who had shown him kindness and generosity: "And he went up, and lay upon the child, and put his mouth upon his mouth, and his eyes upon his eyes, and his hands upon his hands; and he stretched himself upon him; and the flesh of the child waxed warm" (2 Kings 4:34).

And what good deed on Aron's part would have merited such miraculous healing? I learned that there were many. Several years after surviving the death camps of Poland, Aron was a young father living outside of Tel Aviv. As he was riding on his motorcycle one day, he saw a large poisonous snake approaching a little girl and poised to strike. Aron gunned the engine and raced toward the girl, putting himself in the path of the snake. The girl was saved, but the snake bit Aron on the ankle. He was rushed to the hospital and saved by the timely injection of anti-venom. But even as he recovered from the snakebite, Aron was sickened from receiving too much of the life-saving antidote. He languished for weeks in the hospital in a weakened state before recovering completely. The Talmud teaches that saving a single life is like saving the world. Aron had saved a life at the risk of his own. For this alone he deserved to be healed.

Nearly a year after Aron's recovery, I received an invitation to his eighty-fifth birthday party. On the way to the party my wife wondered aloud how atypical it was for me to even consider attending the life event of a patient. In the small town where my grandfather had served as doctor, it had been common and even expected for patients to extend invitations to such occasions. But for a psychiatrist, accepting such invitations is usually considered a violation of appropriate boundaries between doctor and patient. For Aron, however, I made an exception. Never in my career had I witnessed such an amazing recovery, a return from the precipice of death. I still marvel at how Aron was not only healed but also seemed better than before, as if the hands on the clock of time had been moved a few beats backward.

Seeing Aron sitting and beaming at the head of the table, surrounded by family and friends and being feted on such a happy occasion, was a wondrous experience for me, a true moment of joy. He thanked me again and extolled what he described as my life-saving role, but I honestly felt that I was the one who needed to express gratitude. I was one small part of a transcendent chain of events, a messenger sent on a preordained mission. In every doctor's life there should be at least one such moment of satisfaction, one shining opportunity to witness the miraculous glory of healing the seemingly incurable. I witnessed the words of the Psalm 92:15 spring to life: "They will still be fruitful in old age; vigorous and fresh they will be." This was my moment, and I shall never forget it.

As my wife and I got up and prepared to leave the birthday party, a stream of Holocaust survivors in attendance approached us. Each one, in turn, rolled up his or her sleeve and pointed out the numbers tattooed on one forearm, permanent reminders of the evil that they had survived. And each survivor, in turn, expressed the same sentiment: "This person," each one said, gesturing to Aron, "this was a person to save."

Not all older individuals will have such happy endings. Many times there will be little that can be done, and the results will seem tragic. But that doesn't mean we have to give up and cast fate to the wind. Sometimes our very presence is life saving when imbued with a sense of commitment and caring. At other times, as with Aron, our desires for an individual's return to health will help us to take critical steps to actually achieve that goal. After all, we harbor these deep hopes for the health and sustenance of ourselves and our loved ones. We should want nothing less for all our elders.

Lessons from Fire

Place of fire,
place of weeping,
place of madness—

—ZELDA, "PLACE OF FIRE"

The red-hued bricks that run along Piedmont Street do not give up their secrets easily. Dredged from shallow pits south of Boston, the alluvial clay that makes up these bricks is mixed, molded, and then fired in kilns up to 1,800 degrees Fahrenheit, where it is transformed from a soft, pliable material into its hardened final form. These bricks are then trucked to Boston and laid down in soft sandbeds, where they run like a petrified vasculature through the historical walkways and side streets of the city, pooling and clotting in courtyards and municipal plazas. Their worn, rough red faces bring a sense of history to the city.

The bricks along Piedmont Street have a sad history hidden beneath them, a lesson of fire and grief imprinted by the fleeing shoes and charred skin of victims and the steaming rubber boots of firefighters that came together at this spot on the evening of November 28, 1942. Shortly after 11 PM a great and tragic fire erupted in the basement of the Cocoanut Grove nightclub, and within minutes the flames burst furiously up the stairwell and then exploded through the shocked and panicked crowd of revelers packing the renovated speakeasy. Tens of diners dropped at their seats, instantly overcome by the toxic fumes. Hundreds of other women and men—many of them soldiers on pass—died in the stampede to the revolving door in the front of the club, which was rendered useless by the crush of bodies. The fire grew quickly to five alarms as Boston's finest tried desperately to save those individuals trapped by a building riddled with fire code violations. Hundreds of firefighters, police officers, doctors, nurses, social workers, passers-by pressed into service, and, eventually, undertakers worked throughout the night and ensuing days to attend to the survivors and then bury the 492 men and women who had lost their lives. It was the second deadliest single building fire in U.S. history. Amazingly, there is no monument on this spot today, only a parking lot and a small parting of the bricks where a bronze plaque in the sidewalk reminds pedestrians of the event.

The legacy and lessons of the fire, however, revolutionized building safety codes. They also inspired a Harvard psychiatrist by the name of Dr. Erich Lindemann to study the process of acute grief. What happens to someone who experiences such a tragedy? Lindemann asked. How does grief manifest and change over time? His observations were published in a now-classic paper in the *American Journal of Psychiatry* in September 1944. "At first glance," Lindemann began, "acute grief would not seem to be a medical or psychiatric disorder in the strict sense of the word but rather a normal reaction to a distressing situation." But such grief is of great interest to the clinician who wants to understand its vicissitudes and learn to reckon the limits of normality.

Lindemann reported several key observations about grief that we now accept as obvious but at the time had not been documented in any systematic way. He spoke of the sense of unreality that grips the mourner, accompanied by waves of somatic distress, sighing and exhaustion, and mental preoccupation with the deceased, sometimes associated with profound guilt. Morbid grief reactions may appear weeks, months, or even years later, often in distorted ways. For example, Lindemann cited one man who suddenly came down with a grief reaction twenty years after the loss of his mother, triggered, it was believed, when he reached her age at the time of her suicide. Other individuals adopt characteristics, even illnesses, of a deceased loved one or continue to function, but in a "wooden and formal way" devoid of emotion or strong interest.

For both the survivors and the rescuers of the Cocoanut Grove fire, the psychological trauma had the potential to produce its own symptomatic picture, what we commonly refer to today as a post-traumatic stress reaction. Aside from the physical trauma of burns or wounds, the subjective trauma can be equally or even more devastating. The intensely frightful, life-threatening event was a fundamental contradiction to how its witnesses viewed the world. As psychologist Jon Allen describes, such a trauma "may shatter the assumptions that the world is meaningful and benevolent, and that the self is worthy." But the trauma of a terrible fire can at least bring some answers to its victims—a revelation of highly flammable décor, faulty wiring, and locked exits. Trauma resulting from the actions of evildoers is more problematic. For survivors of war or genocide, the search for some theodicy that explains either the silent presence or the glaring absence of God may prove elusive. Worse, the work of evildoers may beg a twisted explanation, where "the most perniciously traumatic result is profound shame and guilt, a sense of oneself as evil."

Old age brings unique perspectives to loss and trauma. It is itself a trauma to many, where the inexplicable and inexorable dissolution of body and mind contradict our view of the world as "meaningful and benevolent." It is also a fundamental challenge to the sense of self, and many elders accept and even adopt ageist views of themselves as useless and decrepit. At the same time, the older mind carries within it newly recognized strengths, including the remarkable ability to adapt to enormous change and trauma, in part by filtering out negative emotions and selectively engaging in more positive activities and states of mind. In old age, survivors of great traumas from earlier in life can teach us how they sustained themselves following unimaginable losses and then went on to thrive.

I have learned from my patients that the crucial antidote is hope. And hope, defined here, goes beyond the mere desire for a better time of life. It goes beyond any rationale that explains the ways of the world, accounts for the mysteries of aging or evil, or explains the nature of God. It is a primal force woven out of both mind and heart that carries us through even the worst of conflagrations. Hope, in this sense, is formed in life's first attachment and is reactivated in all subsequent trusted attachments to others. Too often we imagine that these attachments drop one by one in old age, that they are no longer necessary or even sought. But I have seen the opposite. This is a lesson, among several others, taught by some of the most impressive survivors I have known—those now-aged individuals who survived the Holocaust.

✳✳✳

The forest still stands, but the people are gone. Only a stone memorial guards their place, surrounded by tall grasses that hide bits of ash and bone deep beneath their roots. In this spot on February 4, 1942, more than 920 Jewish men, women, and children from the town of Rakov in what is now Belarus were rounded up by Germans and herded into the town's synagogue. Several shrieking children were stabbed with bayonets and thrown over the heads of the weeping Jews just before the doors and windows were sealed and the building was doused with kerosene. An unspeakable scene of wailing ensued as the once vibrant Jewish community was annihilated in the fire. My patient, now ninety-eight, still weeps when he describes witnessing this horror from a hidden perch in a tree. He gasps audibly when he recalls watching his father being pummeled by a German soldier before he was thrust into the doomed crowd.

When this survivor first told me his story, I was speechless. He held tight to my arm, and I imagined myself as the branches of the tree that supported him during this trauma. I was now a witness. As his psychiatrist I am obliged to ease his suffering, but no medicine of mine can touch such a memory. I have tried hard to understand how he and others managed to mentally survive such traumatic experiences. These aging Holocaust survivors, in particular, have taught me what I have come to call "lessons from fire."

Lesson one is the most difficult for a doctor: *Sometimes the perpetual sadness of many older survivors is not to be healed but shared.* Over time, as memories fade and the voices of lost loved ones grow quieter, all that remains is a closely guarded sadness, persisting as a substitute for the losses. Any attempt to ease this emotion may be a threat to the painful but beloved remnants of memory. What some survivors seek is not medicine or therapy but the attentive presence of a doctor and others to serve as the next generation of witnesses.

Lesson two brings a paradox: *Surviving a grueling trauma does not inoculate a person against the stresses of aging.* A patient once told me that the small daily indignities she faced in the nursing home felt worse than her experiences in a Siberian labor camp. I realized that she could not bear feeling a victim again, even in small measure.

Lesson three gives me hope: *Survivors of great trauma can sometimes find healing when they give to others what they need themselves.* One patient, a survivor of Auschwitz, recently lost her husband of sixty years. She came to me severely depressed, with thoughts of suicide. I asked her, "How did you have any hope in the camp, knowing that each day could be your last?" She smiled briefly and told me a story: "My dear doctor, I believe in God, and He was with me in the camp. But I also had several young women from my town with me in the barracks. When we had to stand at attention for hours, we stood together, propping up one another when weak. When we dug ditches, we did it together, one holding and moving the arms and shovel for another who didn't have strength that day. We were desperate, but never alone." I referred her to a social club we had created for older people with mild memory problems, and one day I crept into the room during a discussion group and hid behind the corner to listen. One woman spoke disparagingly of her memory: "I am losing my mind," she said. "It is so painful." Then I heard my patient respond in a resolute voice, "You must have hope. We are all in the same boat here, together." As I listened, I could feel the tears welling up in my eyes, but I kept myself hidden, afraid to let the group see their doctor weeping. From my hiding place I witnessed a beloved patient begin to heal herself.

These lessons from fire are not the only points of clinical knowledge that a doctor needs to work with aging victims of trauma, but they're a good start. When facing the last generation of Holocaust survivors, I offer my presence as a doctor and I feel strengthened by their words. "Faith—I still have faith," I hear a survivor say. "Doctor, hope for me!" another commands. These are the primal gifts of life that we share.

The Seamstress

"There is nothing more you can do for me. It is time to die."

These are troubling words for a doctor. They challenge the root mission to heal disease or, in the very least, to relieve suffering. It is at these moments that I have often witnessed colleagues become less scientific and more moralistic with patients, urging them to hang in there and live or to accept some form of hospice care as they are dying. My patient Emma, who spoke these words to me, was not, however, suffering from an imminently terminal illness. Instead, she *felt* terminal in her own eyes. I frequently encounter similar older patients in my work who refuse treatment, believing that it is futile. Such attitudes risk provoking sufficient fear and confusion in both doctor and caregivers that they come to silently agree with the older, despairing individual.

Emma was my patient for nearly ten years, and she lived alone in an assisted living facility for all of that time. At the age of ninety-eight she first expressed to me her wish to die. My progress note from our meeting began the way all my notes on Emma did: "This is a 98-year-old woman with a history of recurrent depression, anxiety, and post-traumatic stress disorder. She survived the Holocaust but lost her husband and children in German concentration camps."

The not-so-subtle message was that her psychiatric illness must be considered within the context of her surviving an almost unspeakable tragedy. I hoped that all clinicians who read my note would pause before seeing Emma, notice her sorrow, and accord her a few extra minutes of time and attention. I also wondered whether other clinicians who encountered her might become consumed, as I sometimes did, in amazement at her survival and horror at her losses.

Emma was a vital young wife and mother prior to World War II. She worked as a seamstress in a small town in Czechoslovakia and lived with her husband and their three young children, ages six months to six years. When the war broke out and persecution of Jews began to accelerate, the family escaped to Antwerp, Belgium, hoping to find a safe haven for their young children, including a fourth child born shortly after they arrived. Eventually, Emma's husband was arrested, never to be seen again. She knew that her own survival was precarious, so she placed the children in a Catholic orphanage that agreed to hide them. She was later arrested by the Germans and spent the next five years in various concentration camps, eventually ending up in Auschwitz. After surviving a death march from Auschwitz and being liberated by American troops, Emma returned to Belgium on foot, only to discover that her children were no more, having been seized by the Germans and sent on a transport to certain death. She wandered around Antwerp "like a crazy woman," she told me, ill and battered physically and psychologically from the death camps and mourning the loss of her entire family. She was later arrested because she had no papers to prove her identity.

And then a small miracle happened. While in jail, she was notified that her youngest son, Chaim, had survived! Emma learned that in 1940 members of the Belgian underground had managed to pull several children out of a cattle car shortly before it left for a death camp. Chaim, then eighteen months old, was small enough to be extracted through an opening formed by several broken planks in the train's siding. Emma's older three children were not so fortunate; they were taken to Auschwitz, where they were gassed immediately on arrival.

Despite her joy over his survival, Emma recounted how it was actually quite difficult being reunited with Chaim, because the seven-year-old boy did not know who she was—he had no memory of anyone in his family—and she was in no shape to be a mother again after her experiences in Auschwitz. She described herself as an inadequate and even abusive mother during their first few years together. Even sixty years later she was consumed with guilt and anguish over her behavior. At times she expressed her own incredulity that the boy returned to her was even her son, although I have seen this grown man and he is her image. When I first met Chaim he told me, quite simply, "It is a miracle that I even stand before you."

Emma related these experiences to me during each monthly appointment, filling the minutes with a long and painful list of losses and trauma, all woven with an unbearable and seemingly unbreakable fiber of depressive and guilt-ridden memories and beliefs. She wept and beat her chest and asked me, "Why? Why?" I listened and offered support, but I had no answers for her. I initially tried to fall back on the pharmacologic moorings of my training, offering her one antidepressant or antianxiety medication after another, but none helped. Most caused dizziness and unsteadiness, which jeopardized her daily walk around campus—the one consistent activity that gave her some peace. And then, after several years of treatment, she informed me that our work had come to an end, that no efforts could overcome her agony.

Despite the great tragedy of her life, Emma at ninety-eight seemed to share a common belief with many old and frail individuals that any and all treatments for despair are futile given their advanced age and overwhelming illness. Multiple blows have taught them that modern medicine can neither slow the process of aging nor alter the inevitability of further decline and death—despite so many claims to the opposite. Even many clinicians have jumped on the bandwagon here, arguing that late-life depression is less "illness" and more a natural reaction to circumstance. As psychotherapist Stanley Jacobson writes, "The high rate of depression among nursing home residents is surely related to the mere fact of their being nursing home residents, immersed in infirmity and impending death." The end result, Jacobson believes, is that clinicians overdiagnose depression, applying a pathological label to what is actually a normal and predictable response to aging. Of course, this argument distorts the true definition of major depression, conflating it with a range of nonpathological states such as sadness and grief. However, we might conclude from this perspective that psychiatric treatment for late-life depression is often a waste of time, a fountain of youth folly no better than so many other spurious claims. I do not think that most clinicians overtly believe this, but many clinicians do hear these doubts from older patients, who in various ways express unremitting despair. In this state a patient's belief in the futility of treatment, regardless of the belief's veracity, can easily become the major barrier to all forms of therapy.

In Emma's case she did not believe that treatment could restore her will to live, because she linked her emotional state with her failing body, the failure of so many past treatments to quell her anguish, and, ultimately, the loss of her young children. And the waters run deep with her because after leaving Europe with her one recovered child, she never loved again, never married, and grew more isolated with time—even from her son and his four children.

Emma's life has been uniquely tragic, but I see bits and pieces of her in so many other older patients. Sometimes pain or immobility or unresolved grief over a dead spouse can consume the entire world of sick and debilitated older individuals, blotting out the possibility of anything other than death to rescue them. Clinicians who hear this and try and fail repeatedly to engage the patient in treatment often come to agree with the futility of treatment, out of frustration, anger, fear of failure, narcissistic injury, or their own despair.

So how does a doctor proceed? One response to an older patient's belief in the futility of treatment is to approach it as a form of suicidal thinking. There is rarely a stated intent or plan to actually commit suicide. Instead, older individuals who lack the energy, will, or physical capability to kill themselves may engage in indirect life-threatening behaviors, such as refusing to eat or drink, take life-sustaining medications, or undergo critical diagnostic tests or treatments. In these circumstances, psychiatric assessment is warranted to identify underlying causes that may yield a variety of treatments. This traditional clinical approach asserts that, even though aging itself cannot be cured, the factors distorting the patient's perspective *can* be treated. Thus, the patient refusing treatment or begging to die may be depressed and hopeless, misinformed, terrified, delirious, under the influence of a substance, or in excruciating pain. Regardless of the factor, patients may be wrong in their belief that treatment is futile because their insight and capacity to think clearly and make decisions are compromised.

This is a particularly important consideration for individuals who have limited insight due to brain damage resulting from stroke, tumor, head injury, or other forms of dementia, such as Alzheimer's disease. For example, individuals with damage to the brain's right hemisphere have impaired recognition and sometimes complete denial of specific neurological deficits or illness, and this may interfere with any sense of concern or urgency for treatment. Frontal lobe injury will also impair insight and judgment in addition to producing impaired abstract thinking, disorganization, disinhibition, or apathy. Put together, these deficits may account for an individual's refusal to consider treatment, either because he or she does not recognize the nature and severity of the disease and the potential benefits of treatment or lacks the motivation to do anything about it.

Unfortunately, when the patient expresses a sense of futility, the doctor may not be far behind. After all, the patient may be correct! A review of the scientific facts of a case may confirm that it is futile to expect improvement. The treatment of potentially reversible factors may carry unacceptable risk or may sustain life without improving its quality. Emma felt depressed and traumatized for sixty years—how could I help her now? Multiple treatments failed. I could not restore her lost children or her capacity to love again. Her lifespan had shrunk to a few more years, at best. What could be gained in that time? Was I willing to put her through treatment that would be coercive and could result in more harm than good?

A good clinician can certainly choose a number of different pathways when dealing with older patients who feel treatment is futile. The clinician can, to a reasonable point, pursue a workup to determine why the patient is refusing treatment and then consider addressing reversible factors. Once this is accomplished, the patient can again be presented with treatment options. But a clinician may agree with both patient and family that further treatment is not reasonable and pursue a less active but still caring approach. With either road, the patient's capacity to make an informed decision must be known. With Emma I was stuck between respecting her wishes, if I believed them to be sincere and rational, or shunting them aside and pushing a more aggressive approach with medications because I doubted her decisionmaking capacity. For many months I remained uncertain of the best plan.

My own bias is that we often give up too early with older ill people because of our own impatience and despair. There is a tendency for even the most caring clinician to begin to with-draw from the person who is preventing fulfillment of the root mission of any clinical practice—*healing*. But there is a counter-point to this tendency. We certainly cannot reverse aging, nor can we effectively treat many of the illnesses encountered in our older individuals. However, we can do something about the concerns that often drive them toward choosing death: loss of autonomy, loss of dignity, and loss of life-affirming activities. These are the factors—not physical pain—that have been cited year after year as the main reasons that a small number of indi-viduals have elected to end their lives under Oregon's Death with Dignity Act. It takes a good dose of hopeful imagination to consider the full potential of older individuals—even at ap-parent endpoints. We cannot give up on them even as they give up on themselves.

Emma's request arrived about the same time a poem crossed my desk by a woman from a similar time and culture as Emma: "All this misery—When will I die?" the poet asks and then con-cludes, "I scorn the hopes of the sun and the promises of blos-soms." Just as I began to anticipate Emma's fading away, another small miracle happened. Arriving suddenly on Emma's doorstep was her eighty-five-year-old sister-in-law, Rachel, who was mourning the recent death of her husband, Emma's brother. I had not known anything previously about Rachel, but here she was, suddenly living with Emma and relying on her to translate because Rachel spoke only Hungarian, Yiddish, and some bro-ken English. Emma became her caregiver, her escort to appoint-ments, and her personal translator with all staff in the clinic and at the assisted living facility. She went to meals and activities with Rachel, advised her on what doctors she needed to see, and supported her through her mourning. In turn, Rachel brought great comfort to Emma. She no longer asked for death. She started coming again to appointments, but with less weeping and less anguish.

During one appointment Rachel told me that she had something important to show me. She pulled from her purse two old, creased, black-and-white photographs. The first photo showed an extended family at a wedding. She pointed to herself in the photo, a smiling figure standing near the bride and groom, surrounded by parents, grandparents, aunts, uncles, and many children. Rachel waved her hand over the photo. "All gone," she said, "all lost." No one in the photograph except Rachel had survived the war. She then turned to the other photo, which showed three perfectly dressed and coiffed children sitting on a park bench next to a young woman. "The momma," she said, and pointed to the figure in the photo and then to Emma sitting beside her. "This is Emma and her children."

I had heard about these children for so long that I was startled to actually see their images. Emma grimaced a bit and said that the photo had been taken so long ago that she could barely recognize herself in it. "What were their names?" I asked. Emma took the photo and pointed to each child: "Yankel, the oldest, then Mendel, named after my grandfather, and then my *maidele* [little girl] Sora." I imagined that a small smile crept on her face as she stared at her lost children, but Emma's reaction was subtle and quiet and did not betray her feelings. "It's time to go, Rachel. Put them away; the doctor has other people to see." They both got up to leave, thanking me for the time, and walked away, one supporting the other. In my own eyes Emma seemed a little steadier, a little more dignified. I wasn't sure what, if anything, I had contributed to her renewal, but my own hope in Emma was certainly restored. It was, in the end, a caring relationship that seemed to offer the best antidote to futility.

※※※

In 2008 Emma celebrated her one-hundredth birthday surrounded by her son, Chaim, his wife, four grandsons and their wives, eight great-grandchildren, Rachel, and a nephew. Seeing the entire family together allowed me to glimpse a small repair in the torn fabric of Emma's life. She continued to live in the assisted living facility near my office, and she witnessed the addition of four new great-grandchildren, bringing the number of her living descendents to seventeen. Rachel remained in the adjacent nursing home, because her memory and ability to speak had deteriorated significantly. Emma could no longer walk, and her failing memory had, ironically, brought her some peace as she no longer dwelled on her lost children. Nevertheless, there was no way, I was certain, for Emma to ever be reconciled with the events of her life. There were no necessary acts of retribution, forgiveness, or even forgetting that would bring sufficient understanding or justice to her losses. Old age allowed her, however, one powerful message: "I am still here." We may argue about whether there is triumph in mere survival or whether the apparent quality or meaning of a person's life must always be entered into the equation. On many days I try to take these measurements in my older patients and do what I can to improve them. When I would see Emma, however, such considerations would drop away, and I would simply marvel at her presence. In late spring 2010, Emma passed away just shy of her one hundred second birthday.

Trees

A magnificent date palm tree stands a few paces outside of my office window. Beholding its thickly ribbed and fern-bearded trunk and majestic crown of fronds, I understand why eighteenth-century Swedish doctor and botanist Carl Linnaeus labeled palm trees the "princes" of the plant kingdom. Like the tree outside my window, Jacobo was a prince of a man—a robust and bearded figure with a perpetual smile. He used to visit me often to teach me Spanish and to talk about his life both before and long after he had fled Cuba. My office was a refuge for him, a bower of books and papers that made him feel at home, as if surrounded by his own library. Over time he even planted parts of himself in my bookshelves with select volumes he brought as gifts. Several years ago he proudly presented me with a copy of his own recently completed magnum opus, *Lógica Transcendente*, the product of decades of deep thought and several years of diligent work in his study. Unlike most of the older men and women who visit me in my office, Jacobo was not a patient; he was my friend.

In my profession such a friendship is not unusual for me, even when the difference in ages spans thirty to fifty years and a generation or two. I still marvel at how both the content of our conversations and the mutual regard rarely betrayed our ages. I had first met Jacobo seemingly by chance—although he would argue that nothing is by chance—during my first year as the psychiatrist at the nursing home. While tending to several consults one afternoon, I walked by the bearded, garrulous figure of Jacobo speaking in an animated tone in Spanish to his daughter. They had arrived that day to visit a beloved family member. We exchanged greetings and sort of tumbled over each other in conversation as I tried in my halting Spanish to welcome him to the "Home," as we called it. Before I knew it, Jacobo had designated himself my personal Spanish tutor, and I suddenly had an eighty-year-old friend with whom to discuss history, religion, and the meaning of life.

Mahogany Tree

The parking lot outside the nursing home in which I work is surrounded by mahogany trees. They appear as sentries along the walkways and parking spaces, with thin, angled trunks, wizened barks, and small-leafed crowns that provide only limited, dappled shade. These trees are young, however, because the mature West Indian mahogany that once grew in abundance throughout South Florida can average up to eighteen feet in circumference and soar to more than seventy feet, earning the moniker "King of the Forest." Most captivating is the woody mahogany seedpod, which from the outside resembles a small brownish-gray potato. Once opened, however, it reveals an intricate, five-chambered array of winged seeds imbued with the rich reddish-brown color that makes mahogany such a desirable wood.

Like these trees, my patients surround and guard the passageways around the nursing home, sharing an outward appearance of frailty but containing within lustrous seeds of history and wisdom that have been spread, year after year, throughout the lives of so many others. I have grown close to these patients, even though the time I know them is short because I lose to death almost as many as I gain each year. They are patients, not friends, although sometimes the lines between can get blurry. This is one unique feature of working with the elderly that every doctor discovers with time. Even when attending to the strictest boundaries in the doctor-patient relationship, the burden of illness and the proximity of death force a special bond with patient and family. At that point small decisions, such as a medication dose or a lab test, can have far-reaching consequences.

In geriatrics, facing the death of so many patients is part of the job. Clinical decisions are often shaped by this reality, as maximal gains from therapies are necessary in minimal time frames. The emotional toll varies, but the loss of a patient who is closer to the line of friend evokes a greater level of grief. I have noticed, however, that the practice of medicine has evolved away from this line, in some ways making it easier to bear these losses. In her book *How Doctors Think*, Kathryn Montgomery describes how medicine has increasingly become a business transaction between strangers; the more objective and scientific it has become, "the more easily it can be commodified, detached from a caring physician, and judged by its 'product,' health." She does not, however, propose a "medicine of friends," despite how attractive the virtue of friendship may be to the doctor-patient relationship. For example, she notes that many physicians value the moments of deep connection with patients and their families that sometimes occur during crises as antidotes to "the alienation and detachment of medicine understood as a science." Although friendship between doctor and patient is a lofty ideal and serves a rhetorical purpose in juxtaposition to a medicine of strangers, Montgomery asserts that such friendships are fraught with risks and ethical concerns.

Instead, as a middle ground Montgomery proposes a "medicine of neighbors": "Neighborliness implies a duty, especially in time of need, but a limited duty that leaves considerable room for both self-preservation and performance above and beyond its call." This proposed metaphor for the doctor-patient relationship is valuable, especially as it stipulates "attention and respect" for patients without the emotions and obligations of friendship, which can be intrusive and burdensome for doctor and patient alike. At the same time, however, the very presence of extant or impending losses, hovering over both doctor and older patient, sometimes demands something more than just a good neighbor.

Apple Tree

During a visit with Jacobo one spring, he appeared tired and depressed. After an hour of conversation, however, he was enlivened, and I felt reassured that all was well. Several weeks passed and I didn't hear from him; I called but got no answer. I persisted, and a weakened voice finally answered the phone: "*Mi amigo, no estoy bien.* I am not well," he told me. I was alarmed and insisted, "Jacobo, I must see you soon!" The next day Jacobo came to my office, unable to walk, with an aide pushing him in a wheelchair. The color was drained from his skin, and he appeared gaunt and exhausted. We barely spoke as I beheld his image. The timelessness of our friendship had suddenly hit the reality of aging, and I knew he was dying. At that moment my friend became my patient, and I quickly made arrangements for Jacobo to go straight into the hospital. Within two weeks Jacobo was gone, drifting off to eternal sleep one morning as his liver shut down from an unknown malignancy. It was a startling departure to me, as I had previously tried to deny that, despite our close friendship, Jacobo's eighty-five years always meant that death was not far off.

And so it was with our friendship, a refuge of time we spent together that was unknowingly and perilously a little way away from the end. Jacobo knew this better than I did. He was an incredibly spiritual man who believed with certainty that God created the world and that it was logic, not just emotion or spirit, that could bring this understanding. But when he once spoke of death to me, it was not logic but pure poetry: "When I die," he offered with a mischievous smile, "perhaps I will be buried close to an apple tree, and I will reach out and pluck a fruit from the branch." I looked at him and chuckled, then reassured us both that there were no trees in the near future. But the image remained in me—this gleaming apple, the symbol of all the worldly knowledge that Jacobo so eagerly sought.

As much as I agree wholeheartedly with Montgomery, I must confess what I, and many of my colleagues, have learned: Sometimes older patients become friends and older friends become patients, either way driven by the nearness of death, which eventually comes, often stealthily, and fells another soul from our practice. We are left as the final witnesses to a life long lived, once full of dreams and memories planted lovingly in this world. This is a special honor, one that grows with time if we are able to hold fast to it:

> *Beloved, gaze in thine own heart,*
> *The holy tree is growing there;*
> *From joy the holy branches start,*
> *And all the trembling flowers they bear.*

Epilogue

In the final act of life my patient Rose taught me about the enduring passions of life. The reason for Rose's sudden decline was unexpected. It was not unusual for a ninety-eight-year-old to stop eating. I see this frequently, and the causes are legion: a broken, painful tooth; persistent, corrosive esophageal reflux; depression; a hidden cancer. The reason for Rose's decline, I learned, was love. She had been deeply in love with another man on her floor in the nursing home and had craved and reveled in the affection he provided. When a younger woman of eighty-eight moved onto the unit, Rose's boyfriend broke up with her and took up with the new resident. Rose demanded to know whether this new woman was somehow prettier or feistier, and she begged him to return—to no avail.

The following week Rose had a fit at the bingo game, screaming at her former boyfriend and calling the new woman a whore. In her fury she swept the bingo cards and chips off the table with wild, flailing movements of her arms. All that the staff and other residents could see in Rose was a woman out of control: a bitter, jealous, and belligerent woman who required, many argued, a heavy dose of sedation. Rose took to her room and stopped eating and drinking. She refused all of her medications. When I met with her, she hissed at me and insisted that I allow her to die. Her family was embarrassed and exhausted by her behavior and counseled us to respect her wishes. Several days later she slipped away, taking with her, I hoped, not a feeling of scorn but a last memory of a joyful kiss. Rose's last days might seem tragic, expressions of all the wretched indignities of old age, but I marvel not at the life lost but at the love lost. Even at ninety-eight she had been able to love so deeply that the loss of that love broke her heart.

※※※

In the final act of life my ninety-five-year-old patient Naomi taught me about the preciousness of memory. At the time of her admission to the rehabilitation unit, Naomi was suffering from short-term memory loss, mild delirium, a complete loss of her independence, and a recent hip fracture that rendered her unable to walk. I was asked to see her because every morning she insisted on attempting the same death-defying feat of trying to leave her wheelchair and walk unassisted, despite the pleadings and admonitions of her therapists.

Prior to our appointment I heard Naomi in the hallway crying out in pain and confusion: "Why am I here, Doctor?" she inquired. When we spoke, I tried to reassure her, but she struggled to understand who I was and what I could do to ease her suffering. When I asked about her past, however, she appeared soothed as she related to me many fond memories—her last and most treasured possessions. I leaned in close and smiled at Naomi. "Please tell me about your *most* precious memory, the one memory that stands above them all." "Oh, Doctor," she cooed, "that's easy. I once danced with *Fred Astaire*." My eyes widened, and the disheveled and decrepit-appearing old woman in front of me suddenly lit up like a celebrity. Many years ago, I learned, she and her husband had had a special friendship with Fred Astaire and Ginger Rogers and had spent countless enchanting evenings with the couple. "Tell me, what was it like to dance with Fred Astaire?" I sincerely wanted to know. Naomi seemed to swoon for a moment as a confident, starry-eyed expression rippled across her face. She seemed lost in the memory. "To dance with Fred Astaire, well, that was . . . *heaven*."

❈❈❈

In the final act of life my patient Benjamin taught me about hope. When I first met him, Benjamin was cradling an infant boy in his lap, his slender, bony fingers gently supporting the head and neck. Though his blind eyes could not see the form of his great-grandson below, he felt it, the pride radiating out in the rays of tears that ran down his cheeks. He appeared to me like a proud vintner holding up a prized cluster of grapes to the beaming sun. I knew Benjamin well, as I knew his daughter and granddaughter—all patients at one time. In my work with them I was able to see the lines of development across all three generations—an entire life cycle laid before me.

There is a tendency to compare youngest and oldest generations, in effect infantilizing our most aged and debilitated citizens by assigning them the same expectations for incapacity and dependence. And why not? In appearance and behavior many severely demented individuals closely resemble young children. At least they appear this way to the eyes of someone much younger. But Benjamin was no infant. He had lived for ninety-six years and was still living, despite the loss of much of what had seemed to define him in the past—his memories, his wife, his ability to walk, and his vision. But at the meeting of man and infant, I saw Benjamin in a new light.

I could see the communion of hope between Benjamin and his new great-grandson as it was developing in the infant and ripening in the elder, guiding each from moment to moment. I also saw a more mature form of trust in Benjamin, one that afforded him a sense of tranquility even as his diminishing vision and memory untied him from his past. In other ways he was very much in tune with something much larger than himself, as in the hours he spent in the arts studio running his hands over the wet clay that he would mold into countless shapes. He had an understanding of life that I could not touch—a feeling of closeness to something beyond. In this light the final act of life brings maturation, not just regression. It is a blessed height poorly imagined by the young, but one, in the words of Erik and Joan Erikson, where "the view stretches out its releasing display, and the sky and the clouds perform their slow and gracious maneuvers."

For Rose, Naomi, Ben, and the many other individuals whom I have described in this book, I am reminded that when we see only the silent darkness of old age, we miss the million sparks of life still present. As the poet Zelda writes:

> In the morning, I thought:
> "Life's magic will never return,
> it won't return."
> Suddenly in my house, the sun
> is a living thing,
> and the table with its bread—
> gold.
> And the flower and the cups—
> gold.
> And the sadness?
> Even there—
> radiance.

I began this book by telling how the place where I work as a doctor for the elderly is sometimes called a waiting room for God. It is certainly a place, for those who believe, where a sacred presence hovers close by those in the final stage of life, waiting, hoping, and carrying with it a reconnection with the force that bore us. As T. S. Eliot writes:

> In my beginning is my end. In succession
> Houses rise and fall, crumble, are extended,
> Are removed, destroyed, restored, or in their place
> Is an open field, or a factory, or a by-pass.

Old stone to new building, old timber to new fires,
Old fires to ashes, and ashes to the earth.

This house of God for the elderly is sometimes a house of pain and of loss. But it is also a house of holies, where aging has the potential to be much more than even our imaginations have conceived. For Abraham Heschel, "Just to be is a blessing. Just to live is holy." These words show me where the story of aging begins and where it ends. The final act for all of us is to listen to our elders. "Hope for me, Doctor," my older patients often ask. I turn to them and answer, "I will try my best. Hope for me, too."

Acknowledgments

I share the ancient sentiments of Socrates, who said, "I enjoy talking with very old people. They have gone before us on a road by which we, too, may have to travel, and I think we do well to learn from them what it is like." The origins of this book, then, must be traced to the myriad older relatives, friends, and patients who have been part of my life. They are too numerous to name, but I owe them my deepest gratitude. I was fortunate to grow up with four grandparents who left indelible imprints on my life and work and without whom this book would never have been possible: Simon and Eva Cherkasky and Tany and Etta Agronin. Their vital presence defied all the stereotypes of growing old that I have explored in this book.

Becoming a geriatric psychiatrist does not happen by accident, and the role in which I have encountered the patients described in this book was inspired and nurtured by numerous colleagues. Two psychiatrists, friends, and mentors from Yale Medical School who first inspired me toward psychiatry were Alan Siegal and Dan Oren. My medical school anatomy partners who joined me in the trenches and who also happen to be two of my closest friends are Jimmy Levine and Steve Ugent. During my psychiatric residency at McLean Hospital, Harvard Medical School, I learned to thrive as a young psychiatrist alongside my closest friends Stuart Anfang and Richard Herman. Gabe Maletta and William Orr were two wonderful supervisors during my geriatric psychiatry fellowship at the Minneapolis VA Medical Center. Gabe Maletta helped to secure several critical interviews for this book and continues to be a particularly important mentor in my career. Our work together as editors of our textbook *Principles and Practice of Geriatric Psychiatry* has been a true joy.

The main setting for much of the book is the Miami Jewish Health Systems (MJHS), where I have been working as the director of Mental Health and Clinical Research since 1999. Only such a unique, beautiful, and enriching setting could motivate me to make the hour-long commute each way down to Miami and back day in and day out to engage in clinical work that feels more like a calling than a job. At MJHS I have had the privilege to work with so many incredibly talented individuals who serve tirelessly to improve the lives of the elderly, and I am grateful for their presence. MJHS would not have become such an amazing place—including Florida's largest nursing home at its center—without the unparalleled leadership for more than fifty years of Irving Cypen, known to all of us at MJHS as simply the "Judge," and his wife, Hazel.

I am indebted to Daniel Carlat for reaching out to me on several occasions to do writing projects that led to many of my current endeavors, including this book. I am equally indebted to my former editor at McMahon Publishing, Donald Pizzi, who gave me my first opportunity to write regular columns for several trade publications that eventually formed the basis for this book. Kate McDuffie of the American Association for Geriatric Psychiatry has also worked closely with me as both an editor and a supporter for several writing pieces that are central to this book.

It was my agent, Rafe Sagalyn, who helped, more than anyone, to sculpt the conception for this book out of many ideas and who has been steadfast in his guidance and encouragement. He introduced me to John Radziewicz at Da Capo Press, the most superb editor and mentor I could ever imagine. I also want to thank numerous Da Capo/Perseus staff members who were instrumental in getting the book in shape and then delivered to a wide audience, including Lissa Warren, Kevin Hanover, Lindsey Triebel, Jonathan Crowe, Annie Lenth, and Josh Berman. I was extremely fortunate to have Jan Kristiansson as my copy editor. Rita Jacobs gave generously of her time to read the manuscript and offer detailed suggestions.

Having the opportunity to interview so many individuals for this book was a true honor. I gratefully acknowledge Senator George McGovern, Leonard Hayflick (who went above and beyond the call of duty in reviewing my depiction of his work and the science of aging), Gene Cohen, Sophie Freud, Bernard Lown, Sherwin Nuland, Julie Newmar, Sue Bloland, Diana Eck, Dorothy Austin, Rose and Paul Svarc, Sharon Lee, Bill and Gloria Cherkasky, Rudy and Arlene Cherkasky, James Hutson, Tom Hutson, Herta Neuman, Sandy Cohen, Susan Wohl, Joseph Goelz, Dr. Walter Richardson, Gerald Charness, Marilyn Goldaber, Alfred Friedman, and Mac Seligman.

In addition to those already cited, a good number of individuals have been extremely helpful in discussing many of the issues and cases in this book, including Stephen Scheinthal, Michael Silverman, Robert Bergman, Elliot Stein, Eli Feldman,

Mairelys Martinez, Victoria Barnett, Rita Gugel, Chrystine Kopscik, Fred and Shuli Stock, Leslee Geller, Dana Ryder, Steve Cypen, Alan Cherkasky, Lynn Cherkasky, Ben Colonomos, Jared Weinstein, Shyla Ford, Alice Sarfati, Michael Brodie, Michele Fiorot, Daniel Ghelman, Patricia Jaegerman, Niurka Colina, Jorge Riveros, Rafael Mestre, Jean Kramer, Mark Samuels, Neal Foman, Michael Druckman, Alan Bauer, Amiel Levine, Melba Canals-Hooten, Stephanie Willis, Elizabeth Andrews, Blaise Mercadante, and Leslie Cedar. Up until his premature passing in the fall of 2009, Gene Cohen was extraordinarily generous with his time and interest, and his own work stands as a pillar in the halls of my profession.

I am grateful to so many friends and family who have rallied around me as this book has moved from an idea, to a proposal, and then to its final form. My parents, Ron and Belle Agronin, and my in-laws, Fred and Marlene Lippman, continue to be my greatest inspiration for what life should be after middle age. My siblings and their families all took close interest in the book, especially in helping to come up with a title, and I thank them all: Mike, Ellen, Joni, David, and Lucy Agronin; Robin, Greg, Sarah, and Shayna Druckman,

There is only one way that this book came into fruition, and that is due to the endless love, support, suggestions, critiques, and patience of my wife, Robin, and my sons, Jacob, Max, and Sam. My three boys took acute notice of my frequent attempts over the past few years to sit in solitude in my office writing this book. Despite my best efforts, however, they would undauntedly encircle my bower of books and papers, leap on me like tigers, extort presents and favors for any mention of them in these pages, and lovingly drag me to their respective dens. May I always be blessed with their constant interruptions! In my ongoing journey into the heart of growing old, I will always observe the lesson of aging exemplified by the most successful elders among us: Hang on tightly to the people we are blessed to have in our lives! Henry Wadsworth Longfellow expresses this sentiment so well in "The Children's Hour" as he reflects on his own children's nightly raids:

I have you fast in my fortress,
And will not let you depart,
But put you down into my dungeon
In the round-tower of my heart.

And there will I keep you forever,
Yes, forever and a day,
Till the walls shall crumble to ruin,
And moulder in dust away.

I invite all readers to read my blog and post comments or send e-mails via my website: www.marcagronin.com.

NOTES

❋❋❋

INTRODUCTION

4   **"bony landmarks":** Taken from the Yale Medical School anatomy instruction manual, circa 1987.

5   **"repulsive formaldehyded body":** Bernard Lown, *The Lost Art of Healing* (Boston: Houghton Mifflin, 1996), 74.

6   **"midsaggital cut":** Yale anatomy manual.

7   **"gomers":** Samuel Shem, *The House of God* (New York: Dell, 1978), 38.

8   **"ageism":** Butler defined ageism as "a process of systematic stereotyping of and discrimination against people because they are old" in his Pulitzer Prize–winning book *Why Survive? Being Old in America* (Baltimore, MD: Johns Hopkins University Press, 1975), 12.

9   **a cure for aging:** Aubrey de Grey, with Michael Rae, *Ending Aging: The Rejuvenation Breakthroughs That Could Reverse Human Aging in Our Lifetime* (New York: St. Martin's Griffin, 2007), 8.

9   **age-centric perceptions:** Lars Tornstam, *Gerotranscendence: A Developmental Theory of Positive Aging* (New York: Springer, 2005), 2. Tornstam talks extensively about how societal views of aging are distorted by the age-centric views of younger individuals.

PART I   WHAT IS OLD?

epigraph John Updike, "Endpoint" in *Endpoint and Other Poems* (New York: Knopf, 2009), 4.

HEAVEN CAN'T WAIT

18   **the psychologist's fallacy:** William James, *The Principles of Psychology* (1890; repr., New York: Classics of Psychology and Behavior Sciences Library, 1988).

19   **"opportunity no less":** Henry Wadsworth Longfellow, "Morituri Salutamus: Poem for the Fiftieth Anniversary of the Class of 1825 in Bowdoin College," in *The Poems of Henry Wadsworth Longfellow*, ed. Louis Untermeyer (New York: Heritage Press, 1943), 434.

24 **the family's debt:** Tom Verkuilen, "Cherkasky Lived the Life of 'Family Doctor'" (letter to the editor), *Appleton Post-Crescent*, June 19, 1997.

AGE I MUST

31 **"two paths":** Marc Agronin, "Exploring the Mysteries of Aging: An Interview with Member Gene Cohen," *Geriatric Psychiatry News*, September–October 2009, 5.

34 **"molecular disorder":** Leonard Hayflick, "Biological Aging Is No Longer an Unsolved Problem," *Annals of the New York Academy of Science* 1100 (2007): 6.

37 **Thomas Jefferson captured:** Thomas Jefferson to John Adams, August 1, 1816, in *Familiar Medical Quotations*, ed. Maurice B Strauss (Boston: Little, Brown, 1968).

38 **"really bad for us":** Aubrey de Grey, with Michael Rae, *Ending Aging: The Rejuvenation Breakthroughs That Could Reverse Human Aging in Our Lifetime* (New York: St. Martin's Griffin, 2007), 32.

38 **fundamental causes of aging:** Aubrey de Grey, "Old People Are People Too: Why It Is Our Duty to Fight Aging to the Death," *CATO Unbound*, December 3, 2007, www.catounbound.org/2007/12/03/aubrey-de-grey/old-people-are-people-too-why-it-is-our-duty-to-fight-aging-to-the-death/.

38 **"Depression of Spirits":** Jonathan Swift, *Gulliver's Travels* (London: Penguin, 2003 [1726]), 209.

39 **nine hundred years?:** Diana Schaub, "Ageless Mortals," *CATO Unbound*, December 5, 2007, www.cato-unbound.org/2007/12/05/diana-schaub/ageless-mortals/.

39 **"through natural selection":** Daniel Callahan, "Nature Knew What It Was Doing," *CATO Unbound*, December 10, 2007, http://www.cato-unbound.org/2007/12/10/daniel-callahan/nature-knew-what-it-was-doing/.

39 **"Senescence escorts us":** Schaub, "Ageless Mortals."

40 **"representation of human aging":** Thomas R. Cole, *The Journey of Life: A Cultural History of Aging in America* (Cambridge, UK: Cambridge University Press, 1992), xxi.

41 **disease and disability:** James F. Fries, "Aging, Natural Death, and the Compression of Morbidity," *New England Journal of Medicine* 303 (1980): 10–135.

41 **hardiness of their reproductive systems:** Thomas T. Perls, "The Oldest Old," *Scientific American* 272(1) (1995): 70–75.

41 **cope better with stress:** Marirosa Dello Buono, Ornella Urciuoli, and Diego De Leo, "Quality of Life and Longevity: A Study of Centenarians," *Age and Ageing* 27(2) (March 1998): 207–216.

41–42 **less genetic susceptibility:** Thomas T. Perls, "Centenarians Who Avoid Dementia," *Trends in Neurosciences* 10 (October 27, 2004): 633–636.

42 **"like a minefield":** George E. Vaillant, *Aging Well: Surprising Guideposts to a Happier Life from the Landmark Harvard Study of Adult Development* (Boston: Little, Brown, 2002).

44 **"Human freedom and vitality":** Cole, *The Journey of Life*, xxv.

LONG TIME DEAD?

49 **"full of death":** Ronald Blythe, *The View in Winter: Reflections on Old Age* (New York: Harcourt Brace Jovanovich, 1979), 29.

50 **"Overselling Depression":** Stanley Jacobson, "Overselling Depression to the Old Folks," *The Atlantic Monthly*, April 1995, 46.

54 **doctors held unique esteem:** For a cogent discussion of the changing societal views of doctors, see Richard Horton, "What's Wrong with Doctors," *New York Review of Books*, May 31, 2007, 16–20.

55 **decisionmaking prowess:** Malcolm Gladwell, *Blink: The Power of Thinking Without Thinking* (Boston: Little, Brown, 2005).

56 **illness involves "uncertainty":** Karen Montgomery, *How Doctors Think* (New York: Oxford University Press, 2006), 191; Jerome Groopman, *How Doctors Think* (Boston: Houghton Mifflin, 2007).

57 **"a presumed culprit":** Groopman, *How Doctors Think*, 149.

59 **"uncertainty sometimes is essential":** Ibid., 155.

PART II   OLD AGE ROUNDS

epigraph   Gary Miranda, "Going," in *Listeners at the Breathing Place* (Princeton, NJ: Princeton University Press, 1978), 14.

ISAAC, ERIK, AND ISAK

70 **"the incredible paradox":** Sue E. Bloland, "The Power and Cost of a Fantasy," *The Atlantic*, November 1999, 61.

73 **a no-man's-land:** Sigmund Freud, "On Psychotherapy," in *The Standard Edition of the Complete Psychological Works of Sigmund Freud*, ed. and trans. James Strachey (London: Hogarth, 1964 [1905]), 7: 264.

74 **"period of increased vulnerability":** Erik H. Erikson, "Reflections on Dr. Borg's Life Cycle," in Erik H. Erikson, ed., *Adulthood* (New York: Norton, 1978), 5.

75   **Erikson's eighth stage:** Erik H. Erikson, *Childhood and Society*, 35th anniversary ed. (New York: Norton, 1985 [1950]), 269.

77   **writing projects were "erratic":** Lawrence J. Friedman, *Identity's Architect: A Biography of Erik H. Erikson* (Cambridge, MA: Harvard University Press, 1999), 457.

77   **"death's door is open":** Erik H. Erikson, *The Life Cycle Completed*, extended ed. with new chapters by Joan M. Erikson (New York: Norton, 1997), 113.

78   **mental burdens of caregiving:** Sue E. Bloland, *In the Shadow of Fame: A Memoir by the Daughter of Erik H. Erikson* (New York: Viking Penguin, 2005), 205.

78   **"sustain this deception":** Ibid., 205.

79   **"neither depressed nor bewildered":** Erikson, *The Life Cycle Completed*, 4.

82   **"an incomparable representation":** Erikson, "Reflections on Dr. Borg's Life Cycle," 3.

82   **"not a regret":** Ibid., 2.

86   **"or meaningfully end":** Erikson, *The Life Cycle Completed*, 62.

ANNABE, BARTLEBY, AND THE DOCTOR WHO FLUNKS AGING

90   **intriguing short stories:** Herman Melville, "Bartleby," in *Billy Budd and Other Tales* (New York: New American Library, 1961), 103–140.

91   **"forlornest of mankind":** Ibid., 123.

95   **"unendurable existence":** Henry A. Murray, "Bartleby and I," in *Endeavors in Psychology: Selections from the Personology of Henry A. Murray*, ed. Edwin S. Shneidman (New York: Harper and Row, 1981), 487.

95   **"principle of self-sovereignty":** Ibid., 491.

95   **"the Bartleby complex":** Ibid., 497.

96   **"kings and counselors":** Melville, "Bartleby," 139–140.

96   **"speed to death":** Ibid., 140.

96   **"Ah, humanity!":** Ibid.

96   **the "sick role":** Talcott Parsons, *The Social System* (New York: Free Press, 1951).

JOSEPH RED HAIR

108   **a sense of empathy:** Howard E. Book, "Empathy: Misconceptions and Misuses in Psychotherapy," *American Journal of Psychiatry* 145(4) (1988): 421.

109   **"attainability of fervent wishes":** Erik H. Erikson, *Insight and Responsibility* (New York: Norton, 1964), 118.

109   **"indispensable virtue":** Ibid., 111.

Old Pickled Brain

116   **"all mental phenomena":** John Searle, *Minds, Brain, and Science* (Cambridge, MA: Harvard University Press, 1984), 18.

118   **underlying bipolar disorder:** Bipolar disorder is a psychiatric illness characterized by recurrent episodes of depression and/or mania. Mania is characterized by a persistently and abnormally elevated or irritable mood along with three or more of the following symptoms: hyperactivity (including states of agitation), grandiosity, decreased sleep, pressured speech, racing thoughts, distractibility, and an excessive engagement in reckless or promiscuous behaviors. Common psychotic symptoms associated with episodes of severe mania include delusions (false, fixed beliefs involving jealousy, grandiosity, or paranoia), hallucinations (false perceptions, usually of an auditory or a visual nature), and grossly disorganized thinking or behaviors. More detailed descriptions of bipolar disorder can be found in the official diagnostic manual of the American Psychiatric Association, *Diagnostic and Statistical Manual of Mental Disorders, Fourth Edition, Text Revision* (Washington, DC: American Psychiatric Association, 2000), also known as the *DSM-IV-TR*.

122   **"your ability to recover":** Jay Neugeboren, "Meds Alone Couldn't Bring Robert Back," *Newsweek*, February 6, 2006, 17.

The Strange but True Case of Dawson da Vinci

135   **crucible for schizotypal personalities:** Theodore Millon, *Disorders of Personality: DSM-IV and Beyond*, 2nd ed. (New York: Wiley, 1996), 613.

136   **"somewhat 'crazy' ways":** Ibid.

136   **become more entrenched:** I have described such outcomes in two papers: Marc E. Agronin, "Personality Disorders in the Elderly: An Overview," *Journal of Geriatric Psychiatry* 27(2) (1994): 151–191; and Marc E. Agronin and William B. Orr, "Personality Disorders in a Geriatric Psychiatry Outpatient Clinic," in American Association for Geriatric Psychiatry, ed., *Abstracts, Annual Meeting, March 8–11, 1998, San Diego, California* (Bethesda, MD: American Association for Geriatric Psychiatry, 1998).

137   **even obsessive-compulsiveness:** For a more detailed discussion, see Richard A. Zweig and Marc E. Agronin, "Personality Disorders in Late Life," in Marc E. Agronin and Gabe J. Maletta, eds., *Principles and Practice of Geriatric Psychiatry* (Philadelphia: Lippincott Williams and Wilkins, 2006), 449–469.

PART III   MEMORY

epigraph Joseph Skibell, *A Blessing on the Moon* (Chapel Hill, NC: Algonquin Books of Chapel Hill, 1997), 256.

IF I FORGET THEE

143 **two dotted nostrils:** See Denise Grady, "Self-Portraits Chronicle a Dissent into Alzheimer's," *New York Times*, October 24, 2006, www.ny times.com/2006/10/24/health/24alzh.html?_r=1&ex=1162616400& en=66feba45095d0e0e&ei=5070.

148 **"effervescent reservoir":** Aharon Appelfeld, *The Story of a Life* (New York: Schocken Books, 2004), v.

148 **"imagination sailed":** Ibid.

149 **held the promise:** Robert Butler, "The Life Review: An Interpretation of Reminiscence in the Aged," *Psychiatry* 26 (1963): 65.

150 **"formal operations":** Jean Piaget, The Early Growth of Logic in the Child (New York: Norton, 1969). For a succinct review of Piaget's theory, see Stanley I. Greenspan and John F. Curry, "Extending Jean Piaget's Approach to Intellectual Functioning," in Benjamin J. Sadock and Virginia I. Sadock, eds., *Kaplan & Sadock's Comprehensive Textbook of Psychiatry*, 8th ed., vol. 1 (Baltimore, MD: Lippincott Williams and Wilkins, 2005), 528–540.

150 **"wisdom":** For a particularly rich summary of postformal thinking, see Judith Stevens-Long, "Adult Development Theories Past and Future," in Robert A. Nemiroff and Calvin A. Colarusso, eds., *New Dimensions in Adult Development* (New York: Basic Books, 1990), 125–169.

150 **"such retrospective despair":** Erik H. Erikson, *The Life Cycle Completed*, extended ed. with new chapters by Joan M. Erikson (New York: Norton, 1997), 113.

151 **fact struck me:** Sophie Freud, *Living in the Shadow of the Freud Family* (Westport, CT: Praeger, 2007). All quoted excerpts are from this book.

156 **"time's typhoon":** Sophie Freud, "The Old Woman and Time," *LLI Review* 4 (Fall 2009): 77.

157 **"a point in space":** Henry David Thoreau, *Walden* (1854), www.the concordwriter.com/Thoreau Quotes.html.

SAVANT, OF SORTS

159 **"photographic memory":** www.goodreads.com/quotes/show/67855.

160 **"savant syndrome":** www.optimnem.co.uk. This is the official website of Daniel Tammet.

161 **regular cognitive exercises:** Sherry L. Willis, Sharon L. Tennstedt, Michael Marsiske et al., "Long-Term Effects of Cognitive Training on Everyday Functional Outcomes in Older Adults," *JAMA* 296 (2006):

2805–2814; Amarilis Acevedo and David A. Loewenstein, "Nonpharmacological Cognitive Interventions in Aging and Dementia," *Journal of Geriatric Psychiatry and Neurology* 20(4) (2007): 239–249.

163 **"tip-of-the-tongue" experiences:** A. S. Brown and L. A. Nix, "Age-Related Changes in the Tip-of-the-Tongue Experience," *American Journal of Psychology* 109(1) (1996): 79–91.

163 **age-related differences:** Judith A. Sugar and Joan M. McDowd, "Memory, Learning, and Attention," in James E. Birren, R. Bruce Sloane, and Gene D. Cohen, eds., *Handbook of Mental Health and Aging*, 2nd ed. (New York: Academic Press, 1992), 307–337.

STRENGTH IN NUMBERS

165 **meaning of the collective:** James Lipton, *An Exaltation of Larks*, 2nd ed. (New York: Grossman, 1977).

OLD SOLDIERS

169 **"You poor bastards":** Stephen Ambrose, *D-Day, June 6, 1944: The Climactic Battle of World War II* (New York: Simon and Schuster, 1994), 49.

170 **deny the existence:** A neglect syndrome called anosognosia is classically seen after damage to the right posterior parietal lobe.

170 **a whole-brain conspiracy:** Vision and visuospatial impairments stem from damaged occipital and parietal cortices; impairments in attention, etc., from frontal, limbic, and temporal lobe damage.

170 **"anosognosia":** M. J. Babinski, "Contributions a l'étude des troubles mentaux dans l'hémiplégie organique cérébrale (anosognosie)," *Review of Neurology* 12 (1914): 845–847.

170 **hatred for a paralyzed limb:** This syndrome is known as misoplegia.

170 **delusional beliefs:** This condition is known as somatoparaphenia. See P. W. Halligan, J. C. Marshall, and D. T. Wade, "Unilateral Somatoparaphrenia After Right Hemisphere Stroke: A Case Description," *Cortex* 31 (1995): 173–182.

170 **someone else's severed leg:** Oliver Sacks, *The Man Who Mistook His Wife for a Hat* (New York: Summit Books, 1984).

171 **cognitive deficits:** Y. Kashiwa, Y. Kitabayashi, J. Narumoto et al., "Anosognosia in Alzheimer's Disease: Association with Patient Characteristics, Psychiatric Symptoms, and Cognitive Deficits," *Psychiatry and Clinical Neurosciences* 59(6) (2005): 697–704.

MEMORIES, FALSE AND FIXED

173 **two medical texts:** Thomas L. Stedman, *Stedman's Medical Dictionary*, 10th, rev. ed. (New York: William Wood, 1928); James C. Meakins, *The Practice of Medicine* (St. Louis: C. V. Mosby, 1936).

179   **switching the memory:** Capgras syndrome is an example of this type
      of delusion, in which an individual believes that someone familiar has
      been replaced by an imposter.

179   **mistakenly diagnoses:** Brendan A. Maher, "Anomalous Experience
      and Delusional Thinking: The Logic of Explanations," in Thomas F.
      Oltmanns and Brendan A. Maher, eds., *Delusional Beliefs* (New York:
      Wiley Interscience, 1988), 15–33.

180   **qualify as a delusion:** Karl Jaspers, *General Psychopathology*, trans.
      J. Hoenig and Marian W. Hamilton (Chicago: University of Chicago
      Press, 1963 [1913]).

181   **"delusion-like idea":** Andrew Sims, *Symptoms in the Mind: An Intro-
      duction to Descriptive Psychopathology* (London: Baillière Tindall, 1988).

PART IV   WISDOM

The Elders

189   **successful aging:** George E. Vaillant, "Aging Well," *Journal of Geriatric
      Psychiatry* 15(3) (2007): 181.

192   **a new ability to think:** Gene Cohen, *The Mature Mind: The Pos-
      itive Power of the Aging Brain* (New York: Basic Books, 2005), 7.
      See also the chapter "If I Forget Thee" here for more on postformal
      thinking.

192   **"how the thinker participates":** Judith Stevens-Long, "Adult Devel-
      opment: Theories Past and Future," in Robert A. Nemiroff and Calvin
      A. Colarusso, eds., *New Dimensions in Adult Development* (New York:
      Basic Books, 1990), 133.

193   **"the verge of death":** Marcus Cicero, "On Old Age," in *The Basic Works
      of Cicero*, ed. Moses Hadas (New York: Random House, 1951), 140.

193   **"practice of the virtues":** Ibid., 130.

193   **girded with knowledge:** Ibid., 149.

194   **more positive autobiographical recall:** M. S. Kisley, S. Wood, and
      C. L. Burrows, "Looking at the Sunny Side of Life: Age-Related Change
      in an Event-Related Potential Measure of the Negativity Bias," *Psy-
      chological Science* 18(12) (2007): 1113–1119; Q. Kennedy, M. Mather,
      and L. L. Carstensen, "The Role of Motivation in the Age-Related
      Positivity Effect in Autobiographical Memory," *Psychological Science*
      15(3) (2004): 208–214.

194   **self-reported well-being:** A. A. Stone, J. E. Schwartz, J. E. Broderick,
      and A. Deaton, "A Snapshot of the Age Distribution of Psychological
      Well-Being in the United States," *Proceedings of the National Academy
      of Science USA* 107(22) (June 1, 2010): 9985–9990.

194   **"evolving mental maturity":** Gene D. Cohen, "The Geriatric Patient," in Marc E. Agronin and Gabe J. Maletta, eds., *Principles and Practice of Geriatric Psychiatry* (Philadelphia: Lippincott Williams and Wilkins, 2007), 7.

197   **"pattern recognition":** Elkhonon Goldberg, *The Wisdom Paradox: How Your Mind Can Grow Stronger as Your Brain Grows Older* (New York: Gotham Books, 2005), 20.

197   **render judgment:** Malcolm Gladwell, *Blink: The Power of Thinking Without Thinking* (Boston: Little, Brown, 2005).

197   **Nobel Peace Prize:** See Bernard Lown, *Prescription for Survival: A Doctor's Journey to End Nuclear Madness* (San Francisco: Berrett-Koehler, 2008).

202   **critical to successful aging:** Sherwin B. Nuland, *The Art of Aging: A Doctor's Prescription for Well-Being* (New York: Random House, 2007).

203   **one's purpose in life:** See Menachem Mendel Schneerson, "Attaining Sagacity," trans. Eliyahu Touger (Brooklyn, NY: Sichos, 1998).

203   **"the unifying element":** Ibid., 2.

204   **notion of spiritual wisdom:** Abraham Heschel, *The Insecurity of Freedom: Essays on Human Existence* (New York: Farrar, Straus and Giroux, 1967), 77.

204   **"need a vision":** Ibid., 84.

204   **"the horizon of honesty":** Ibid., 78.

204   **"the dignity of old age":** Ibid., 84.

204   **"the attainment of wisdom":** Ibid.

205   **"gerotranscendence":** Lars Torstam, *Gerotranscendence: A Developmental Theory of Positive Aging* (New York: Springer, 2005).

JUST WORDS

211   **language comprehension:** M. Carreiras, J. Lopez, F. Rivero, and D. Corina, "Linguistic Perception: Neural Processing of a Whistled Language," *Nature* 433(7012) (January 6, 2005): 31–32.

212   **true meaning:** See Ray Monk, *How to Read Wittgenstein* (New York: Norton, 2005).

212   **rare form of dementia:** This form of dementia is called primary progressive aphasia; the inability to name things, anomia.

LIAR, LIAR

epigraph Carlo Collodi, *Pinocchio* (New York: Children's Classics, 1987 [1883]), 104.

216   **truthfulness:** Tom L. Beauchamp and James F. Childress, *Principles of Biomedical Ethics*, 5th ed. (New York: Oxford University Press, 2001), 283–284.

218   **"when veracity conflicts":** Ibid., 284.

218   **"Frank but not blunt":** Ibid.

219   **many are relieved:** B. D. Carpenter, C. Xiong, E. K. Porensky et al., "Reaction to a Dementia Diagnosis in Individuals with Alzheimer's Disease and Mild Cognitive Impairment," *JAGS* 55(3) (2008): 405–412.

219   **this form of truth-telling:** James F. Drane, *Becoming a Good Doctor: The Place of Virtue and Character in Medical Ethics*, 2nd ed. (Kansas City, MO: Sheed and Ward, 1995), 55.

PART V   A MILLION SPARKS

epigraph   Grace Schulman, "Celebration," *The Atlantic*, May 2009, 64.

FINAL ACTS

epigraph   Marcus Cicero, "On Old Age," in *The Basic Works of Cicero*, ed. Moses Hadas (New York: Random House, 1951), 158.

233   **"subservient to no one":** Ibid., 140.

234   **"a season ripe for death":** Ibid., 154.

234   **"a 'full life'":** Daniel Callahan and Kenneth Prager, "Medical Care for the Elderly: Should Limits Be Set?" *Virtual Mentor* 10(6) (June 2008): 404–410, http://virtualmentor.ama-assn.org/2008/06/oped10806.html. See also Daniel Callahan, *Setting Limits: Medical Goals in an Aging Society* (Washington, DC: Georgetown University Press, 2003).

236   **timeless responsibilities:** Cicero, "On Old Age," 152.

MENDED

242   **normal pressure hydrocephalus:** Cerebrospinal fluid (CSF) is the clear, alkaline liquid that bathes and cushions the brain within its cranial vault. Hydrocephalus—sometimes called "water on the brain"—results from an abnormally increased volume of CSF. NPH represents a chronic, insidious form of hydrocephalus.

LESSONS FROM FIRE

epigraph   Zelda, "Place of Fire," in *The Spectacular Difference: Selected Poems*, trans. Marcia Falk (Cincinnati, OH: Hebrew Union College Press, 2004), 147.

250   **acute grief:** Erich Lindemann, "Symptomatology and Management of Acute Grief," reprinted in *Sesquicentennial Supplement to the American Journal of Psychiatry* 151(6) (1994): 155.

252   **"shatter the assumptions":** Jon G. Allen, *Coping with Trauma: Hope Through Understanding*, 2nd ed. (Washington, DC: American Psychiatric Publishing, 2005), 290.

252   **"profound shame":** Ibid.

253 **an unspeakable scene:** A documented account of the destruction of the Jews of Rakov during World War II can be found at these websites: www.eilatgordinlevitan.com/rakov/rakov.html; http://horwitzfam.org/histories/Rakov%20Belarus%20Report.doc; and www.eilatgordin levitan.com/volozhin/vol_pages/vol_gb_archive_03.html. A photograph of the stone memorial to the murdered Jews of Rakov can be found at www.eilatgordinlevitan.com/rakov/rakov.html.

THE SEAMSTRESS

259 **"high rate of depression":** Stanley Jacobson, "Overselling Depression to the Old Folks," *The Atlantic*, April 1995, 47.

263 **Death with Dignity Act:** See Department of Human Services, Oregon, "Oregon's Death with Dignity Act: The First Year's Experience," February 18, 1999, http://oregon.gov/DHS/ph/pas/docs/year1.pdf; and Department of Human Services, Oregon, "Eighth Annual Report on Oregon's Death with Dignity Act," March 9, 2006, http://oregon.gov/DHS/ph/pas/docs/year8.pd.

263 **"promises of blossoms":** Zelda, "All This Misery—When Will I Die?" in *The Spectacular Difference: Selected Poems*, trans. Marcia Falk (Cincinnati, OH: Hebrew Union College Press, 2004), 61.

TREES

267 **magnum opus:** Jacobo Forma, *Lógica Transcendente* (Kearney, NE: Morris, 2006).

269 **a business transaction:** Kathryn Montgomery, *How Doctors Think* (New York: Oxford University Press, 2006), 177.

270 **moments of deep connection:** Ibid., 181.

270 **"medicine of neighbors":** Ibid., 185.

272 **"the holy branches":** William B. Yeats, "The Two Trees," in *The Rose* (1893; repr., Whitefish, MT: Kessenger, 2004), 24.

EPILOGUE

276 **a blessed height:** Erik H. Erikson, *The Life Cycle Completed*, extended ed. with new chapters by Joan M. Erikson (New York: Norton, 1977), 128.

277 **"'Life's magic'":** Zelda, "Ancient Pines," in *The Spectacular Difference: Selected Poems*, trans. Marcia Falk (Cincinnati, OH: Hebrew Union College Press, 2004), 177.

278 **"ashes to the earth":** T. S. Eliot, "Four Quartets" (1943), www.tristan.icom43.net/quartets/coker.html.

278 **"Just to be":** Abraham J. Heschel, *The Insecurity of Freedom* (New York: Farrar, Straus and Giroux, 1967), 82.

Selected Bibliography

※※※

One of the greatest joys of reading any book is that you never know where it will take you. For any such journeys into the realm of aging prompted by this book, a complete bibliography would be enormous and beyond the scope of the present effort. I therefore refer readers first to the numerous notes in the text to learn more about specific topics that I discuss. However, I would be remiss not to recommend the works of several individuals whom I have relied on to teach me both the basics and the minutiae of aging.

I am a student of the life cycle as it unfolds into later life, and I believe that the work of Harvard professor and fellow psychiatrist George Vaillant has laid the foundation for much of what we know about this process. He has built on the work of Erik Erikson, Daniel Levinson, and others to provide some of our most contemporary perspectives, and he is able to weave them into fascinating case studies. I recommend that the reader begin with the following work:

George E. Vaillant, *Aging Well: Surprising Guideposts to a Happier Life from the Landmark Harvard Study of Adult Development* (Boston: Little, Brown, 2002).

Standing shoulder to shoulder with Dr. Vaillant is Gene Cohen, one of the founding fathers of geriatric psychiatry. As

I describe throughout the book, he has taken the earlier work of Erikson and others and integrated aspects of both modern neuroscience and positive psychology. I was extremely fortunate to get to know Gene before his untimely death in late 2009. I wholeheartedly refer the reader to two of his books:

Gene D. Cohen, *The Creative Age: Awakening Human Potential in the Second Half of Life* (New York: Avon Books, 2000).

Gene D. Cohen, *The Mature Mind: The Positive Power of the Aging* Brain (New York: Basic Books, 2005).

For more detailed, historical accounts of aging, I always turn to the work of Thomas Cole:

Thomas R. Cole, *The Journey of Life: A Cultural History of Aging in America* (Cambridge, UK: Cambridge University Press, 1992).

Thomas R. Cole and Sally Gadow, eds., *What Does It Mean to Grow Old? Reflections from the Humanities* (Durham, NC: Duke University Press, 1986).

For books that provide inspiring, positive perspectives on aging, I recommend the following:

Wayne Booth, *The Art of Growing Older: Writers on Living and Aging* (Chicago: University of Chicago Press, 1992).

Barbara Myerhoff, *Number Our Days: A Triumph of Continuity and Culture Among Jewish Old People in an Urban Ghetto* (New York: Simon and Schuster, 1978).

Sherwin B. Nuland, *The Art of Aging: A Doctor's Prescription for Well-Being* (New York: Random House, 2007).

Mary Pipher, *Another Country: Navigating the Emotional Terrain of Our Elders* (New York: Riverhead Books, 1999).

Lars Tornstam, *Gerotranscendence: A Developmental Theory of Positive Aging* (New York: Springer, 2005).

There are a number of excellent books that cover not only the science of aging but also the fascinating story of the search for immortality. Without question one of the best was written by award-winning author Jonathan Weiner:

Jonathan Weiner, *Long for the World: The Strange Science of Immortality* (New York: HarperCollins, 2010).

Several other excellent books that cover the territory include the following:

Aubrey de Grey, with Michael Rae, *Ending Aging: The Rejuvenation Breakthroughs That Could Reverse Human Aging in Our Lifetime* (New York: St. Martin's Griffin, 2007).

Stephen S. Hall, *Merchants of Immortality: Chasing the Dream of Human Life Extension* (Boston: Houghton Mifflin, 2003).

S. Jay Olshansky and Bruce A. Carnes, *The Quest for Immortality: Science at the Frontiers of Aging* (New York: Norton, 2001).

Thomas T. Perls and Margery Hutter Silver, with John F. Lauerman, *Living to 100: Lessons in Living to Your Maximum Potential at Any Age* (New York: Basic Books, 1999).

A more specific (and one of the best!) book on wisdom is this one:

Elkhonon Goldberg, *The Wisdom Paradox: How Your Mind Can Grow Stronger as Your Brain Grows Older* (New York: Gotham Books, 2005).

For those interested in larger societal issues on aging, the key source is unquestionably Robert Butler, one of the founding fathers of the field of geriatrics, who, sadly, passed away in the fall of 2010:

Robert N. Butler, *The Longevity Revolution: The Benefits and Challenges of Living a Long Life* (New York: PublicAffairs, 2008).

To learn more about Erik Erikson and his theory of the life cycle, I refer the reader to Lawrence Friedman's outstanding biography as well as to the other selected works listed here:

Sue Erikson Bloland, *In the Shadow of Fame: A Memoir by the Daughter of Erik H. Erikson* (New York: Viking Penguin, 2005).

Erik H. Erikson, *Childhood and Society*, 35th anniversary ed. (New York: W.W. Norton & Company, 1985 [1950).

Erik H. Erikson, *The Life Cycle Completed*, extended ed. with new chapters by Joan M. Erikson (New York: Norton, 1997).

Erik H. Erikson, Joan M. Erikson, and Helen Q. Kivnick, *Vital Involvement in Old Age* (New York: Norton, 1986).

Lawrence J. Friedman, *Identity's Architect: A Biography of Erik H. Erikson* (Cambridge, MA: Harvard University Press, 1999).

Finally, for readers who themselves work in the field of aging and are interested in books that provide details on the science of aging and on how to work successfully with older patients, I refer them to the following books, including several of my own:

Marc E. Agronin, *Alzheimer's Disease and Other Dementias*, 2nd ed. (Philadelphia: Lippincott Williams and Wilkins, 2008).

Marc E. Agronin, *Therapy with Older Clients: Key Strategies for Success* (New York: Norton, 2010).

Marc E. Agronin and Gabe J. Maletta, eds., *Principles and Practice of Geriatric Psychiatry* (Philadelphia: Lippincott Williams and Wilkins, 2007). A second edition is due out in 2011.

Colin A. Depp and Dilip V. Jeste, *Successful Cognitive and Emotional Aging* (Washington, DC: American Psychiatric Press, 2010).

Leonard Hayflick, "Biological Aging Is No Longer an Unsolved Problem," *Annals of the New York Academy of Science* 1100 (2007): 1–13.

Robert D. Hill, *Positive Aging: A Guide for Mental Health Professionals and Consumers* (New York: Norton, 2005).

S. Jay Olshansky, Leonard Hayflick, and Bruce A. Carnes, "No Truth to the Fountain of Youth," *Scientific American*, June 2002, 92–95.

CREDITS AND PERMISSIONS